Best wishes for a medical career of service and fulfillment.

John P. McGovern, M.D.

Congrats!

John P. McGovern, MD

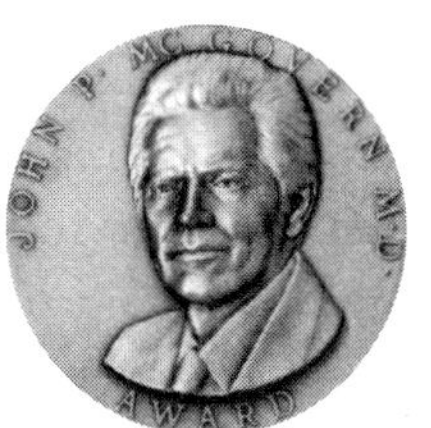

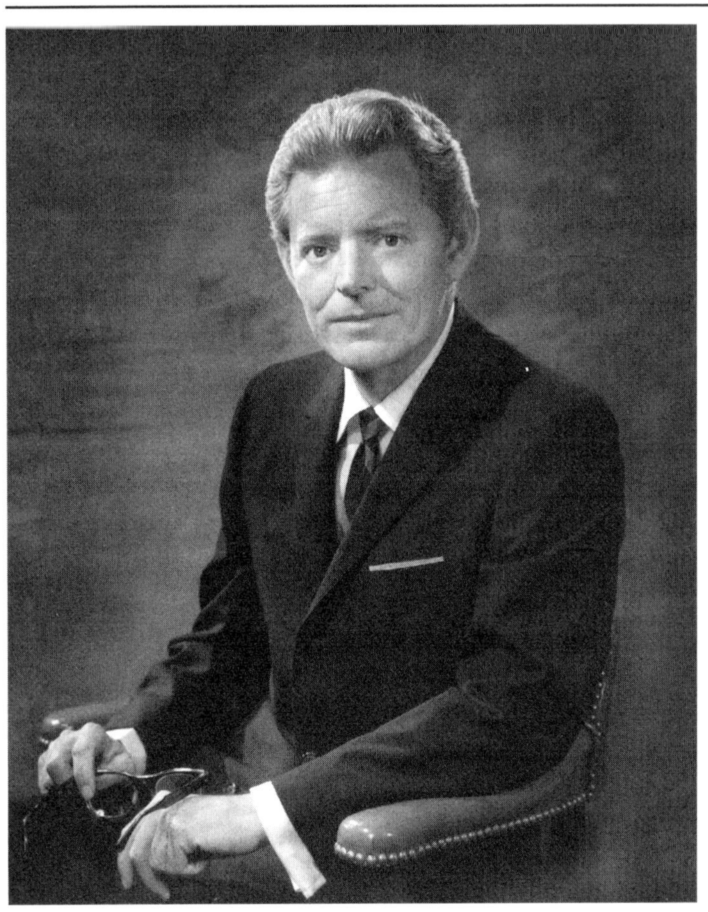

JOHN P. McGOVERN, MD

A Lifetime of Stories

BRYANT BOUTWELL

Foreword by MICHAEL BLISS

TEXAS A&M UNIVERSITY PRESS

College Station

First edition

This paper meets the requirements of ANSI/NISO Z39.48-1992

(Permanence of Paper).

Binding materials have been chosen for durability.

Unless otherwise credited, photographs courtesy of the Texas Medical Center Archives.

LIBRARY OF CONGRESS CATALOGING-IN-PUBLICATION DATA

Boutwell, Bryant.
John P. McGovern, MD : a lifetime of stories / Bryant Boutwell ; foreword by Michael Bliss.—First edition.
pages cm
Includes bibliographical references and index.
ISBN 978-1-62349-122-2 (cloth : alk. paper)—
ISBN 978-1-62349-164-2 (e-book)
1. Pediatricians—Texas—Biography.
2. Allergists—Texas—Biography.
3. Houston (Tex.)—Biography.
4. McGovern, John P., 1921–2007. I. Title.
RJ43.M34B68 2014
618.9200092—dc23
[B]
2013042063

For

Kathrine Galbreath McGovern

Contents

Foreword

McGovern Medical Magic

MANY OF US RECOIL AT THE THOUGHT of mixing idealism and money in medicine. Surely our best students go into medicine to help people, not to get rich. Surely medicine is a vocation, a calling. Its greatest reward is the satisfaction that comes from having served the sick, or, for a researcher, from having added to human knowledge of sickness and health. We do not think that concern for material rewards should be a driving factor in health care. We worry that high principles have a way of dissolving when they are immersed in dollars.

Dr. John P. McGovern, an allergist and immunologist, became fabulously wealthy practicing medicine in Houston, Texas. He did it all the while focusing his life on the highest humanist values. He proclaimed himself a disciple of the great physician Sir William Osler, and the evidence of the biography you are about to read is that Jack McGovern was indeed a great "Oslerian" physician and human being. Instead of selling out his ideals for more dollars, Dr. McGovern reversed the formula. He gave away his dollars to advance his ideals. It was money that proved soluble in idealism. This is a book about one of the most influential medical philanthropists of our time.

The key, as an old pork-packer once said, is to make the best bacon possible and you'll find that profit is one of your by-products. I won't give away any of the terrific stories that Bryant Boutwell, the perfect McGovern biographer, has to tell in these pages. But his main point is this: if you take a young American of boundless energy and eagerness to serve, have a great educator (Wilburt Davison of the Duke Medical School) introduce the lad to Oslerian principles of medicine, plunk him down in a fertile environment (Houston, Texas) in the golden age of modern medicine after 1950, you can sit back and watch his smoke.

Laboring unceasingly at his vocation, Jack McGovern practiced good Oslerian medicine, and for him (as in fact for Sir William Osler himself), a by-product of success was a high income. He then practiced good investing, the by-product of which was even more income. He created a charitable foundation, which has concentrated on using its wealth to supply medical and community and Oslerian needs.

These pages detail the remarkable extent of the McGovern Foundation's work in Houston—its name seems to be everywhere in the awe-inspiring Texas Medical Center—and they also remind us that another of John P. McGovern's significant legacies is the perpetuation throughout the medical world of the Osler name and values. Dr. McGovern himself was one of the founders of the American Osler Society. A fledgling medical fan club when it was formed in 1970, the AOS has become the senior organization in North America devoted to memorializing Osler's life and perpetuating his humanitarian values in medicine. The American Osler Society's philanthropic activities have extended to Osler sites in Canada and Great Britain as well as in the United States.

Because of his frailty, Dr. McGovern had to curtail his public activities in years well before his death. I was very fortunate that he was able to come out for a lecture I gave on Osler at the University of Texas Medical Branch in Galveston in 2001. The occasion was part of the ceremonies marking the creation of the John P. McGovern Academy of Oslerian Medicine on that campus, yet another living monument to the two great physicians.

The Jack McGovern I met that day was a gentle, soft-spoken physician, warm, friendly, and encouraging in the best Oslerian manner. Here, clearly, was a man cut from Osler's cloth. I wish I could have spent more time with him. Fortunately Bryant Boutwell, an accomplished writer and historian, did spend many, many hours with McGovern, and in recent years he has also lived with the McGovern archive and with the memories of people close to his subject. He gives us a rare and well-told story of how high principles in medicine can generate great material success, which in turn can be put to good and lasting use in the best of all causes, serving humanity.

—MICHAEL BLISS

Distinguished Professor Emeritus, University of Toronto

Acknowledgments

I AM PROFOUNDLY GRATEFUL to many people for helping me bring this book to life. At the Houston Academy of Medicine–Texas Medical Center Library and its Historic Research Center, Dr. Maximilian Buja and Deborah Halsted kindly provided me an office in the archives and unlimited access to the library's many fine collections; senior archivist Philip Montgomery, among his many kindnesses and genialities, performed invaluable service as a sounding board for ideas; Alethea Drexler was always available to handle special requests to locate documents and photographs; and M. J. Figard, who manages the McGovern Rare Books Collection, provided support in the research phase of the book. My deepest thanks to them all.

Emily Scott, my research assistant, helped me organize my database and final citations. Likewise, Pam Lewis and Jane Brust, trusted colleagues and outstanding copy editors, took on the task of first reviews and helped immensely with the early draft. Elizabeth White, although she retired in 2008 from her lead role in building the rare books collection with the help of Dr. McGovern, has been a strong support and capable advisor to the author. Her experience of working directly with Dr. McGovern and his beloved collection of rare medical books proved extremely helpful.

At Yale, Dr. Majid Sadigh, then on the faculty at the School of Medicine, generously offered me his basement library for research and writing, and Mark Gentry and the archivists hospitably provided me a special tour of Cushing's rare book and anatomical collections.

Academic reviewers included Dr. Thomas R. Cole, who directs the McGovern Center for Humanities and Ethics at the University of Texas Health Science Center at Houston and provided thoughtful advice and guidance along the way.

Special thanks also go to Michael Bliss, an outstanding historian and a former president of the American Osler Society, who provided feedback and steady encouragement; and to Texas A&M University Press and its editor-in-chief, Mary Lenn Dixon, who showed immediate interest in this project and has been faithful to it throughout. Her support and guidance have been invaluable. Thanks also to Patricia Clabaugh, project manager, who shepherded the manuscript through the production process. Copy-editor Margret Kerbaugh is a first-rate wordsmith and was a pleasure to work with throughout the process of finalizing the manuscript.

Gay Collette and Orville Story, who died during the course of this project, were of great assistance, and they are sorely missed. The author's digitalized interviews with them are preserved in the Texas Medical Center's Historical Research Center. Among the happiest times on this project were two days in 2010 that I spent at Orville's home in Fredericksburg, Texas, with his wonderful wife, Barbara. Glenn Knotts, a friend of many years, died in 2002, but not before sharing with the author priceless stories about McGovern and an understanding of what it was like to keep up his pace.

I also want to thank the faculty and staff of the John P. McGovern Center for Humanities and Ethics at the University of Texas Health Science Center at Houston, particularly Shirley Pavlu and Angela Polczynski, who were heroically patient and supportive as I juggled writing and teaching duties on opposite sides of our medical city.

I thank the membership of the American Osler Society, from whose scholarship and collegiality I have benefited in untold ways.

Finally, enough cannot be said for the confidence and trust that Kathy McGovern has reposed in me or to express my gratitude to her for it. Her support has meant everything to the outcome of this project. I could not have undertaken or sustained it without her blessing. I am indebted also to Kathy's outstanding staff at the McGovern Foundation, including especially Julia Mitchell. The archives I mined for over two years are very much Julia's work.

And my deep gratitude and love go to my wife, Lana, and daughters, Mae, Brittany, and Brooke—all of whom brighten my life beyond measure.

John P. McGovern, MD

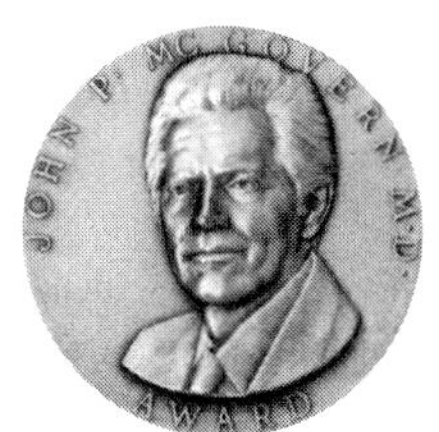

Introduction

IN 1980 JOHN PHILIP MCGOVERN, MD, was honored for his thirty-five years as a physician with the publication of a 680-page festschrift called *Appreciations, Reminiscences, and Tributes Honoring John P. McGovern.*[1] The "big blue book," as it became known, was a collection of tributes written by 229 then-current and former faculty colleagues, students, and friends throughout the United States and the world. Read the book cover to cover, distill the sentiments, and you come to realize this was a much admired man with more than a few friends. Their collective words define him: they termed him "brilliant clinician," "revered professor," "insightful researcher," "prolific author," "skilled administrator," "dedicated medical historian," "dynamic leader of diverse medical organizations," "enlightened scholar," "concerned humanitarian," "gifted speaker," "lifetime student," "loyal friend," and "devoted husband."

John P. McGovern, at age fifty-five, was at the top of his game when his lifelong friend, former Duke pediatrics professor Grant Taylor, first conceived the big blue book. Since graduating from Duke University's School of Medicine in 1945, McGovern had launched a medical career in allergy and immunology and built the nation's largest privately owned allergy clinic. He had trained many of the leaders in his field and set an example of how a patient-centered physician/scientist and man of energy can make a difference. In his spare time he had relentlessly saved and invested his money to build a foundation worth nearly $200 million in his lifetime. It would allow him to continue making a difference for others well into his retirement and beyond.

With the publication of *Appreciations*, McGovern had another thirty-two highly productive years left. He wasted no time. In addition to establishing and nurturing the allergy clinic, during his life in medicine McGovern held 17 professorships, received 29 honorary doctorates (appendix A), authored 252 professional publications, including 26 books in the medical sciences and humanities, and did all of this while serving as president or chief elected officer of 15 professional societies in medicine. He also served as editor or member of the editorial board of more than 20 scientific journals (appendix B) and endowed 29 annual medical award lectureships in universities nationwide as well as at the Smithsonian in Washington, DC (appendix C). The list of national and international awards he received during his lifetime requires a separate appendix for this book (appendix A).

In Houston alone you can visit McGovern Lake and McGovern Children's Zoo, the McGovern Museum of Health & Medical Science, and the McGovern Campus of the Texas Medical Center, or you can dine in the McGovern Commons—and that's just in one part of town.

In Houston's Texas Medical Center, a medical city in and of itself, John P. McGovern's reputation and reach touched all institutions. While such men as Michael DeBakey (Baylor College of Medicine), Denton Cooley (Texas Heart Institute), and R. Lee Clark (the University of Texas M. D. Anderson Cancer Center) built great academic institutions and renowned reputations, McGovern transcended the traditional boundaries of institutional identities and medical specialties. He brought together big institutions, different health professions (medicine, dentistry, nursing, public health, informatics, biomedical research) and provided bold interdisciplinary ideas and a team approach to health care that today is recognized not as just a good idea, but as essential. His outlook was holistic; he always saw the big picture, but without losing track of the parts and how they fit together. He was an inspired and tireless integrator.

I first met John McGovern in 1995 when I was a faculty member and associate dean at the University of Texas Medical School at Houston. A news journalist by original training who first joined the University of Texas M. D. Anderson Cancer Center in the early 1970s, I had come to the Texas Medical Center as a science writer working in M. D. Anderson Cancer Center's Public Information Office, where it was possible to run into important physicians, scientists, and political figures of the day as they came to meet the institution's founding president, R. Lee Clark. Here also were governors, Nobel laureates, presidents of major universities, the members of city and state government, presidents of nations worldwide, even presidents of this nation. As a writer and storyteller I wanted to connect the dots, collect the stories, and know the history of this Disneyland of medicine.

While I knew of John P. McGovern, I did not know him personally in 1995 when I first approached him with the intent to write a book on the history of the University of Texas Medical School at Houston and the Texas Medical Center to honor the school's thirtieth anniversary. I had joined the medical school as a faculty member and assistant dean overseeing communications and community outreach. Such a history was needed and timely, given that most of the deans in our school's history were living and their stories needed collecting.

I pointed out in a brief letter to McGovern that I intended to research and write the book on my own time after work and on weekends and that I hoped to cover all the expenses for the project with outside funds, as a gift to my school. This evidently caught his interest, for he wrote back shortly, agreeing to provide some cautious funding up front from his foundation to support videotaping oral history interviews with each of the living deans.[2]

Within a year the interviews were completed, and I was writing and sending McGovern sample copy. This prompted a telephone call, taken by my assistant, who reported that Dr. McGovern was on the line and it seemed not just urgent but "very urgent." The urgency was to inform me that he not only liked what he was reading, he wondered if he could be co-author on the project. In short order we became collaborators and friends. Our friendship lasted until the end of McGovern's life.

McGovern's beautifully appointed home was located in a luxurious high-rise only a mile from my office. It overlooked the entire Texas Medical Center, as if the building had been purposely placed to give him this panoramic perspective of the medical city below.

Here evening after evening McGovern and I met to talk about the project, and more often than not, we would wind our way into the stories behind the institutions spread out before us, and into the history of medicine in general. I soon learned how much I did not know. A single question on a medical topic could lead to a half-hour dissertation complete with McGovern's historical perspective and footnotes. I was a privileged listener with a unique opportunity to learn directly from a man who had not only

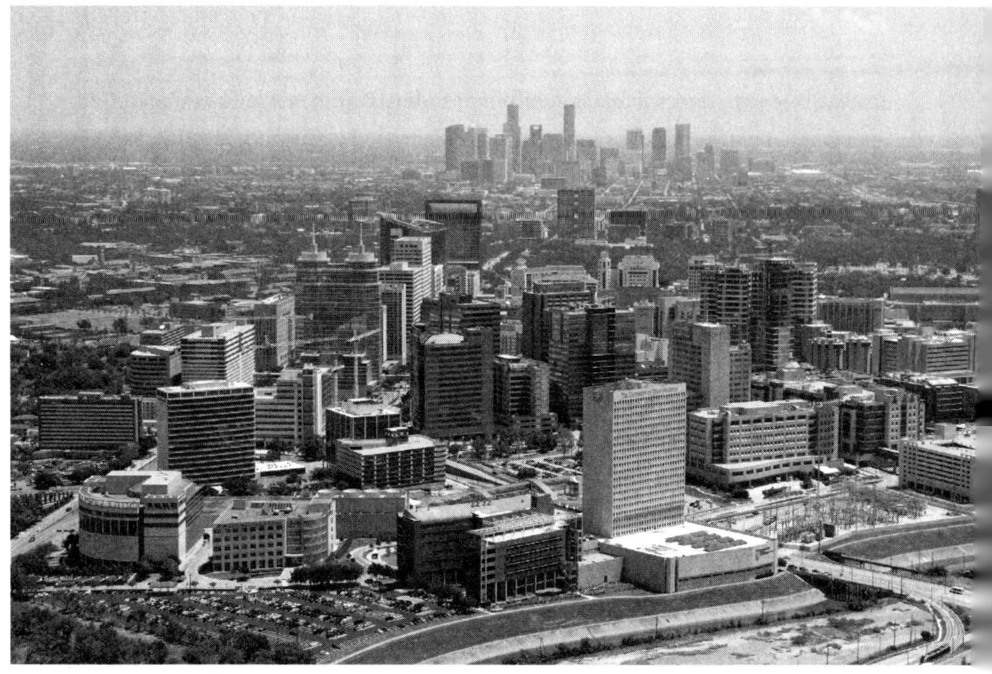

INTRO 1. Aerial photograph of the Texas Medical Center with downtown Houston behind in the distance. Houston has two distinct skylines—one for business and one for health care. *Photo by Dwight C. Andrews.*

lived the history of the medical city that glittered below in the night, but had also shaped much of that history himself. He had a perspective on health care that few in the nation could match. He would tell stories about physicians and medical scientists he had known and would share tidbits from the history of American medicine and the Texas Medical Center. I would tell stories I had gleaned here and there, and hours would fly by unheeded.

My education continued with each visit, and soon one evening a week grew into two or three. Sometimes at the end of a visit McGovern would hand me a book on Sir William Osler and suggest it might be of interest. The relevance of this part of my education was lost on me at the time, but it will become obvious to the reader of this book.

Needless to say, I absorbed everything I could from these conversations. When upon occasion I would have the luck to offer a piece of information new to McGovern, whose mind was encyclopedic, he would sometimes look impressed and other times cock his head doubtfully to the side. Particularly in the latter case, by our next meeting he was likely to have researched my remark and to be ready with either a correction or a compliment, depending on the outcome of his inquiry. In such a way our friendship was born.

As McGovern approached his ninth decade, his ability to remember detail began to fade. The process of our conversations changed to meet his needs. Now he would start a story and would come to dates and names he knew well, but that he could not pry loose from his memory; he would grope for the words, and he often apologized for his "lethologica." The first time he used the term I had never heard it and suspected him of having invented it on the spot. But when I checked I found that lethologica is in fact a documented psychological condition that impedes the ability to recall words. My task now was to fill in those lost names so that he could complete his stories and minimize his lethological frustrations.

In this way, McGovern relived his stories: the stories of Duke Medical School and his beloved dean there, Wilburt Davison; the stories of coming to Houston in 1956 to start an allergy practice and joining such academic enterprises as Baylor College of Medicine and the University of Texas M. D. Anderson Cancer Center (then M. D. Anderson Hospital and Tumor Institute); the stories of international research and leadership at the highest levels of his profession; the stories of his childhood and extended family; the stories of his foundation—in short, the stories of his life.

My role soon evolved from friend and medical history student to writing assistant and editor. In the last decade of his life, McGovern could no longer complete all his book reviews and some other writing he had promised several years earlier. There were books in press that needed his foreword. I volunteered to help, and so my education continued.

I soon learned that I was likely to hear a lecture from McGovern on the importance of any word I tried to edit out for him and of the sentence it appeared in. An assignment to cut thirty words was certain to get three hundred words of verbal pushback, accompanied by documented reasoning—and additional reading if needed. What I thought was a victory at the end of a long evening was often followed by a phone call the next afternoon summoning me to return and try again. Entirely pleased with himself, McGovern would inform me, "I stayed up last night and rewrote the section, so now we need to cut forty words." I could see him smiling through the phone. His first intent was always to make the project of the moment the very best it could be. Good enough was never an option; McGovern had been on a lifelong quest for excellence. But I was well aware that he also enjoyed introducing mischief into a piece of work that he knew I was perfectly content with.

At the conclusion of an evening's work in McGovern's home, we would to push aside the manuscripts and galley proofs, move away from the worktable, and gaze across the room through the floor-to-ceiling window that framed the view of the world's largest medical center below—an immense, vibrant panorama of human drama and medical discovery that never pauses, never rests.

At such times McGovern would occasionally leave medical talk behind and dip into older recollections, his fund of stories from his boyhood. I never took notes during these impromptu sessions, but I had developed an ability over the years to absorb a story as it was told. The stories he recounted to me then come back to life in this book: stories about himself as a child in Washington, DC, where he learned to play marbles—and to play for all the marbles; about his father, a surgeon during the uncertain years of the Great Depression; about his mother and his beloved Granny Brown; about his cousin, the actress Helen Hayes, who was as proud of McGovern as he was of her; about his first seven dollars; and about the foundation he had created with a few thousand dollars that he grew into millions for its beneficiaries.

McGovern spent the last five years of his life sixty miles south of Houston in a Galveston Island beach house that he and his wife Kathy bought to be closer to the sea air and the Gulf breeze that seemed to assuage his failing health. He and Kathy shared a special love of the beach. They had been avid fishermen, wade fishing the salt marshes of the back bays to bring home stringers of speckled trout, redfish, and flounder.

On my pilgrimages to the beach house during these last years, I was regaled with medical history supplemented by fishing stories. I grew up in Mississippi; fishing furnishes my earliest memories and has for many years served as my main weekend pass time away from work. I typically began a visit to the beach house by reeling out a fishing story and displaying photos of my most recent catch, which once included an 8.5-pound trophy speckled trout I had caught just a few miles away. The proof was in a glossy photograph.

McGovern studied the photo in silence for a moment and then confessed, with defeat in his crackling voice, that the biggest trout he had ever caught was smaller by a pound; and that before he could retrieve it for his wall, the taxidermist's shop had burned down. I regretted my bragging and appealed to Kathy for permission to bring the mounted trout from my wall to put in her husband's study facing the beach. Happily, for the next three years McGovern began each day in his comfortable chair with a view of the Gulf of Mexico outside his window and of that magnificent fish soaring across his study wall.

My last visit to see McGovern was a sad one; he could hardly recall my name. Our combined attempt to complete one last story together was not working despite my continued efforts to add the names and dates he could no longer remember. Sensing he was weary, I got up to leave with a heavy heart. The stories he loved so much and wanted to relive were just piecemeal bits, words that fell to the floor without processing. Yet, as I helped him to his unsteady feet, I sensed something different about him. He grabbed my elbow with force and grinned, pointing up to the fish. "See that fish there? Since I started losing my memory, I get away with telling people I caught it myself."

That was classic McGovern, and it lightened a dark day. The fish is now back in my study, along with a framed photo of John P. McGovern watching over it. The sparkle in his eye and that one last broad grin are indelibly etched in my memory.

Within a month of that last visit, I answered a call one Thursday morning on the way to work. McGovern had been hospitalized with pneumonia over the Memorial Day weekend. He was at John Sealy Hospital. I immediately turned my car away from the Texas Medical Center and headed sixty miles south to Galveston. I entered the silent world of his room, where only the noisy pulse of monitors provided any hint of life other than the distraught face of his wife. At my unexpected arrival, Kathy jumped to her feet and told me what the doctors had just told her—that all of the medications in their arsenal had failed, and that this might be her husband's last day.

It was. Within hours he was gone. That restless stream of thought and energy that had been Jack McGovern had left the room. Those left living moved in tearful silence. Outside it was a bright spring day, May 31, 2007, two days short of his eighty-sixth birthday.[3] The birthday card I had mailed just days earlier would be delivered into other hands.

Writing McGovern's biography seems a natural consequence of our friendship. I knew him well. Or, did I know him at all? Who was John P.

McGovern? Was he a saint without faults? What gave him the drive and enthusiasm to take on the huge labors that he completed in one lifetime? How did the history of medicine influence his life, and how did he influence the future of medicine? All these questions deserve attention.

To find their answers I began by visiting the John P. McGovern Historical Collection and Research Center of the Houston Academy of Medicine–Texas Medical Center Library, located a few miles south of the medical center in a nondescript building unnoticed by many who drive past it daily. Here John McGovern, along with many other great leaders—including the founders of the Texas Medical Center—can be found speaking clearly through the papers and mementoes that they have left for others to explore. Here are the voices of the past recalling the stories of years gone by. We can make them out them if we take the time to listen.

At the very beginning of this project, surveying the warehouse-sized collection of archived boxes containing these voices of the past, I naively asked the archivist, Phil Montgomery, which boxes were McGovern's. With the sweep of his hands I learned we were not talking boxes, we were talking floor-to-ceiling rows of heavy-duty industrial shelves where boxes are carefully numbered and stacked two deep. The archivist had prepared an eighty-six-page, single-spaced "finding aid"[4] or inventory of the materials that was still in progress as more items arrived.

With the finding aid to Collection 115 in hand, you can readily explore McGovern's well-lived life. Here are childhood photos, his first report card, his mother's watch, his first passbook savings account, letters to his friend and lifelong mentor Wilburt Davison, and a lifetime of correspondence with medical colleagues around the world. Here in these boxes is the record of his love of medical history and his passion for medical research and discovery.

If you stayed late into the night, who knows but you might even hear his voice.

I would come to learn that these were not all the boxes housing McGovern's archives. Others would appear mysteriously at my door, as if he himself had pushed them forward in the middle of the night.

In my office in the front of the building where researchers come and go, I hung a heavy famed portrait of McGovern that I found waiting on a shelf in the back. It had been a Christmas present from his staff and was dated December 1976. As I worked, my old friend looked down at me, following my journey through the boxes of his life. I began writing his stories under his gaze and with his voice in my ear.

McGovern would not want this book to be a chronological recital of his curriculum vitae. Rather, he would want it to be *stories* about his life providing a historical perspective on events that shaped it, and the backstories that interested him in the paths he chose. With this thought in mind, I have developed this biography.

Early in his life, as you will learn in these pages, young Jack McGovern determined that he wanted to develop a life of service. On interview day at Duke University School of Medicine, he surprised the admissions committee of one, Dean Wilburt Davison, with a clear concept of himself that stood out from all others. He needed only a few words: "I like people and science, and I want to put the two together in service as a physician."[5]

He was accepted by Davison on the spot, and proof of the sincerity behind his statement lies on the pages ahead. McGovern's life of service and his love of people are what this book is all about. It is this writer's hope that those who read it will be inspired with a greater understanding of what one man with immense energy and a laser focus on his goals can accomplish in a single lifetime.

Chapter One

Growing Up in DC

THE YEAR 1921 was a good year to be born.

World War I had ended on the eleventh hour of the eleventh day of the eleventh month in 1918. For the first time in years, America's focus on the war was receding into the past, and many Americans felt that the Great War was the last war. The 1920s, comfortably positioned between the two world wars, was a time of great optimism and growth.

These were the years when F. Scott Fitzgerald was publishing classic chronicles including *This Side of Paradise* (1920) and *The Great Gatsby* (1925). Sinclair Lewis published the Pulitzer Prize-winning novel *Arrowsmith* (1925), about a physician from a small midwestern town, torn between research and community medicine. The Roaring Twenties, the Jazz Age—call it what you will, it was a special time in American history.

It was the time of Prohibition, which tested our nation's morality in new ways as speakeasies and gang violence emerged on a grand scale. A new type of American woman came into her own in this era, one who smoked, drank, danced, and voted. The Great Depression was more than a decade away, and newspaper headlines of the year were reporting such good news as the purchase of twenty acres by the New York Yankees to build Yankee Stadium, the delivery by air of the first US transcontinental mail from San Francisco to New York, the lectures on a new theory called relativity delivered in New York City by a professor named Albert Einstein, and the isolation of a substance called insulin by two scientists at the University of Toronto.[1] A man in England named Churchill was making a name for himself as Minister of Colonies.

Dig deeper into the headlines of 1921, and you find more ominous signs of events to come. Lenin proclaimed new economic politics in Russia, deadly race riots rocked Tulsa, Oklahoma, the Communist Party of China was founded, and Adolf Hitler became the leader of the National Socialist German Workers (Nazi) Party. Still, many of these darker headlines of the day were lost to front pages that had the nation buzzing as Babe Ruth hit his 120th home run on June 10 and became the home run champion of baseball, and then just a month later set a new record of 137 career home runs.

During that month of June in which Babe Ruth was making history, John Philip McGovern was born in Washington, DC. To family and friends, he was Jack.

Of all the good fortune in young Jack's life, perhaps the best was being born into the McGovern family. On June 2, 1921, he became the first (and would remain the only) child of Francis Xavier McGovern (1893–1951) and Lottie Brown McGovern (1893–1979). Welcoming his new child to the world, F. X.—or Mac, as he was really called—sat down and in the strong and artful hand of the general surgeon he was, wrote his son a three-page letter on American Red Cross stationery.

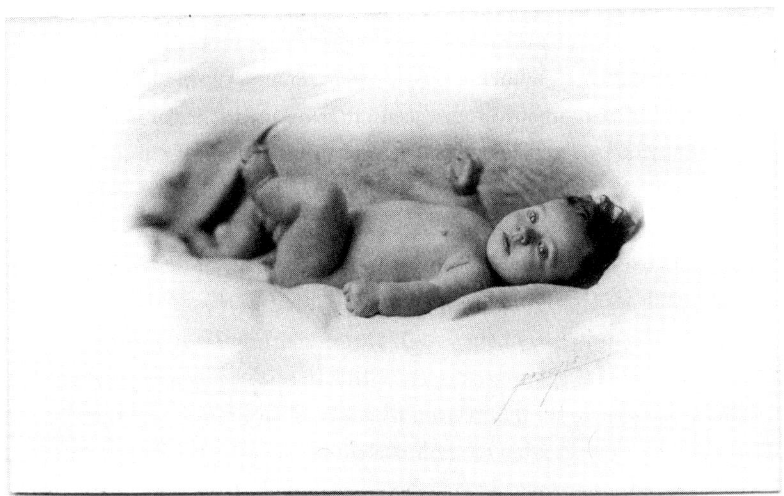

FIGURE 1.1. Jack McGovern, age four months.

My dear Little Jack:

This is your first letter. Daddie wants you to be as good a little boy as you can. You are too young now to know what your Dear Mother suffered in order to bring you into this world, but you will one day know and realize it. You have a dear sweet Mother; a mother who will always love and cherish you. She has shown Daddie by her actions how intensely and sensibly she loves you and I want you always to love her. Never show by actions or word anything but a boy's love for his mother. As you grow older Daddie will tell you of your Dear Mother and he will teach you to love her in a way that will make her realize that all she has done and will do for you will be appreciated by you. Mother will, I am sure, teach you to love Daddie. I love Mother, Mother loves me, we both love you and you love us both. Hence our little family will be happy in love. So Jack my darling Boy, spare your Mother all you can. She has not yet fully recovered from her efforts to bring you into this world and needs all the rest she can get.

With a world of Daddie Love for his Boy,
I am, affectionately
Daddie[2]

Although it rustles with the lively ghosts of Victorian sentimentality, this letter is nevertheless revealing. It promises a close family, with parents who offer much and who expect much. They welcome their new son into their household with a written compact assuring love and requiring it in return. A letter to a beloved newborn suggesting its duty to return love is remarkable, to say the least, and the paternal ethic behind the letter almost certainly suggests an important source of McGovern's ideas about gratitude, which would be expressed later in his philanthropy. Gratitude to family and gratitude to society at large are not at that far a remove.

On the day of their son's birth, both mother and father were twenty-eight years old. Mac McGovern was a proud man, a physician who worked hard as a surgeon for little pay in these years approaching the Great Depression. He was tall and lean, a sharp dresser, with a dapper mustache over a broad grin that his son inherited and used to good advantage all his life.

The very existence today of such early letters suggests the collector that Mac's son would become. The archives of Jack McGovern's lifelong correspondence are measured in linear feet, and they have been invaluable to me in coming to understand and attempting to recreate the remarkable eighty-six years of life that lay ahead. Another of McGovern's collections—rare medical books—now requires an entire section of the Houston Academy of Medicine–Texas Medical Center Library—one of the largest medical libraries in the world.

Francis Xavier McGovern, the surgeon whose son Jack would follow him into the field of medicine, was born December 25, 1893, and grew up in New York, the city of his birth. Francis Xavier's father, Philip McGovern (1855–1912), was born in County Cavan in Northern Ireland and came to the United States with his parents at age five. Philip's wife, Ann Gallagher (1858–1915), was born in New York City. Her parents had also emigrated from Ireland in the 1850s on the heels of the Irish Potato Famine. The two wed in 1882 and produced ten children, two of whom died in infancy. With five brothers and two sisters, Francis was the third youngest of the eight siblings.[3]

Educated in New York City, Mac attended Fordham University, where he took his medical degree in 1915. Perhaps it should be noted that his newly minted surgeon's hands were nearly as adept with a baseball as with a scalpel. A standout on the university's baseball team, Mac would pass along to his son a lifelong love of the sport, as well as the benefit of his exceptional hand-to-eye coordination, which would serve McGovern well in his devotion to baseball and tennis—and, incidentally, to marbles.

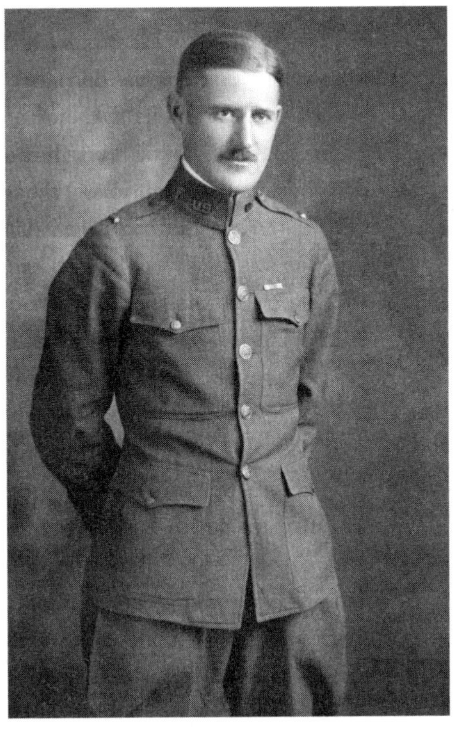

FIGURE 1.2 Francis Xavier McGovern, MD.

On July 4, 1917, just four days after he had completed his internship at Bellevue Hospital, Mac joined the Army Medical Corps and was relocated to Washington, DC, as a member of the US Public Health Service on the surgical staff of Walter Reed Hospital. In Washington he met and fell in love with a native of the city, Lottie Brown. The two wed on October 13, 1918, with Mac's younger brother, the Reverend Albert McGovern, officiating.[4]

In the course of his assignment to Walter Reed, Mac McGovern found himse back in New York City with his new bride, studying infected wounds with Nobel laureate Alexis Carrel. It was Carrel who had pioneered vascular surgery and worked with aviation great Charles Lindberg to invent the first perfusion pump. Later Mac was reassigned to head the surgical staff of the US Public Health Service Hospital in Kansas City, Missouri, before returning to Washington to establish himself in private practice and start a family in the city that would remain home permanently.

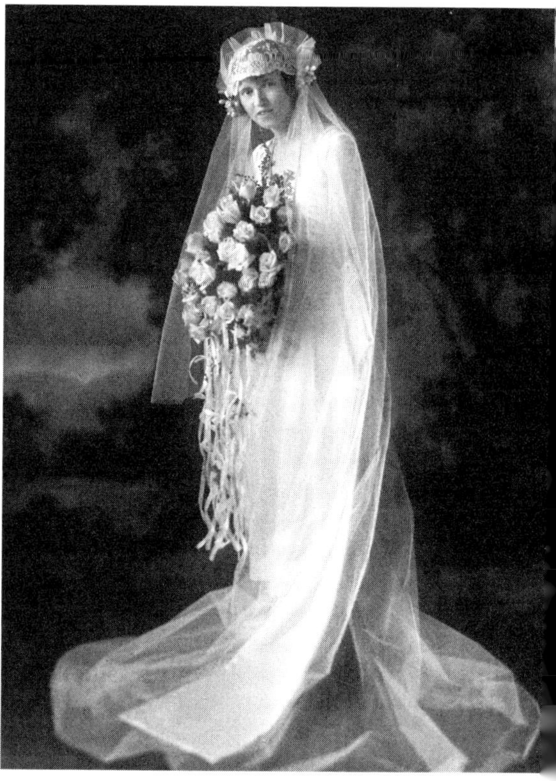

FIGURE 1.3. Lottie Brown on her wedding day, October 13, 1918.

In 1921, the young Washington surgeon found himself back in Walter Reed Hospital, not as a staff surgeon but as a new father. Here Lottie Brown McGovern delivered their child. The delivery, as Mac's letter to the infant McGovern suggests, extremely difficult, with life-threatening implications for the mother. Lottie wo remain bedridden for more than a month afterwards, and any plans for additic children ended.

In Washington, the young family settled comfortably into apartment life at 4 Connecticut Avenue, number 107. To this day, Connecticut remains the beauti tree-lined avenue it was in the 1920s—a major Washington thoroughfare beginn at Lafayette Square across the street from the White House and moving northwes Farragut Square, DuPont Circle, Cleveland Park, Chevy Chase, and points beyor

The McGoverns' apartment, which today would be called a condominium, on the first floor of a six-story brick art deco apartment building at the corne Davenport Street and Connecticut Avenue in the neighborhood of North Clevel

Park. Apartment 107 was small, with one bedroom and one bath, but it was comfortable and affordable, with friendly neighbors and plenty of children to provide a community of belonging for young Jack. With a growing son, the McGoverns eventually moved upstairs to a larger apartment, number 209, with two bedrooms and two baths.

A vacant lot between apartment buildings off Connecticut Avenue provided a convenient and well-worn playground where Jack McGovern and his boyhood friends played ball well into the evening hours, when parents started their dinnertime search. Thomas Mahoney, a childhood friend, said that "this was the meeting place for touch football, baseball, soccer, and other activities we thoroughly enjoyed, without the organization and parental supervision that seems to be required nowadays. Jack's competitive spirit and athletic skills were evident in the manner in which he entered into these games."[5] With a bat clenched in his hands, his blue eyes narrowed on the ball, and his Irish blond hair standing around his head like a bushy nimbus, he would have been an intent, fiercely focused player, determined to win.

Another outdoor sport that Jack loved was fishing, especially with his mother's half-brother, Frank Schweitzer (1874–1965), affectionately referred to by the youngest McGovern as "Brother Frank." And he liked camping out with the Boy Scouts. These pastimes suggest the friendly and outgoing character long remembered by those who knew Jack as a boy, including the hospital staff who often saw the senior McGovern with his attentive son in tow during weekend rounds.

In 1929, as Jack reached his eighth birthday, Mac became a member of the senior attending staff of Washington's Garfield Memorial Hospital, where he established himself as a proficient surgeon known for keeping long hours and for dedication to his patients. His good work earned him wide respect, culminating fifteen years later, in 1944, with the promotion that made him chief of surgery at Garfield and president of the hospital's medical staff.

Garfield Memorial was one of many hospitals in Washington dating back to the Civil War. The hospital was named for President James Garfield, who was assassinated in July 1881 after only four months in office. Designed by John Shaw Billings (who plays a prominent role later in this book), the hospital was built by Adolf Cluss, a friend of Garfield's and an important architect of the day, who also designed the National Museum—the Smithsonian Institution's first museum building—with its recognizable red brick façade. Now renamed the Arts and Industries Building, it remains one of the Washington Mall's most famous landmarks.

Mac McGovern, who had joined the medical staff of Garfield Memorial as the bottom dropped out of the nation's economy, spent fifteen of the twenty-four years of his medical career in this aging public hospital, known for its dilapidated wards. They were overcrowded, sorely outdated, and ill equipped to handle even the local citizens, much less the many war-wounded patients admitted for care. Here, in one of Washington's oldest and busiest hospitals, even the best and most dedicated health-care professionals were challenged by the seemingly endless flood of destitute and hopeless Washingtonians. They were the malnourished and ill who overflowed from the city's famous soup lines during the Depression into overcrowded and ill-funded District hospitals like Garfield.[6]

By July 1, 1932, Washington felt the full brunt of the Depression. Although the District's primary business, the government, escaped collapse, federal salaries were slashed to the bone, many workers were given furloughs without pay, most government departments saw reductions in force affecting a third of the families living in the District, four banks went into receivership, many people lost their life savings, and business throughout the District was crippled.[7]

The statistics are eye-opening, observes historian Robert McElvaine, for "from the top of prosperity in 1929 to the bottom of depression in 1933, the GNP dropped by a total of 29 percent, consumption expenditures by 18 percent, construction by 78 percent, and investment by an incredible 98 percent. Unemployment rose from 3.2 to 24.9 percent. By almost any standard, the United States was in its worst crisis since the Civil War."[8] One can only imagine the impressions made on young Jack, who would have witnessed scenes of desperation and despair on the streets mirrored in the crowded hospital wards where his father worked. Mac was not indifferent to the suffering around him. He is said to have moved a few hundred dollars from his personal savings into a friend's bank in hopes of helping it keep its doors open. The bank unfortunately failed, and the McGovern money was lost.

Headlined events of the day also included the infamous Bonus March in the nation's capital during the spring and summer of 1932, when World War I veterans petitioned for immediate cash payment of their service certificates, bonus payments promised by the government but not redeemable until 1945. More than seventeen thousand veterans and their families camped out in ramshackle huts made from scraps of lumber, canvas, tin cans, and packing cases. At one point more than eighty thousand people (one hundred thousand by some estimates) joined the protest.[9]

By July 28, 1932, orders were given to General Douglas MacArthur to clear the camps and the remaining ten thousand protestors.[10] The flames of the makeshift shelters burned into the night as protestors fled in mass panic, leaving a bewildered nation trying to understand such ruthless action. Jack McGovern was only eleven years old, and these international headlines from his own city were scored into his childhood memory.

As hospitals filled with the destitute and the malnourished, paychecks at Garfield Memorial were repeatedly cut. But Jack would tell the *Houston Chronicle* in a feature interview in 1996 that he never once heard his father complain during these hard times, although as a surgeon he was "the last one to be paid." He also recalled among friends that his father often returned from the hospital during the Depression years having been paid with a family's homegrown garden vegetables or a freshly plucked chicken. Both were equally welcomed into his mother's kitchen.[11]

Mac had other important lessons to teach his young son. Physicians, he believed, should care not only about their own practice, but also about the profession at large. In 1933 Mac McGovern deepened his commitment to the Medical Society of the District of Columbia and proved himself through a multitude of committee assignments. In 1938 he was named chairman of the new executive board, a position he held until 1942.[12] His colleagues remembered him as a tireless leader of the District's medical society, one who would always go into battle for his principles, even when that meant taking on tough challenges. One such challenge was to address the growing need to close the many small and outdated Civil War hospitals like Garfield Memorial and consolidate them into one large, state-of-the-art facility capable of meeting the District's future needs.

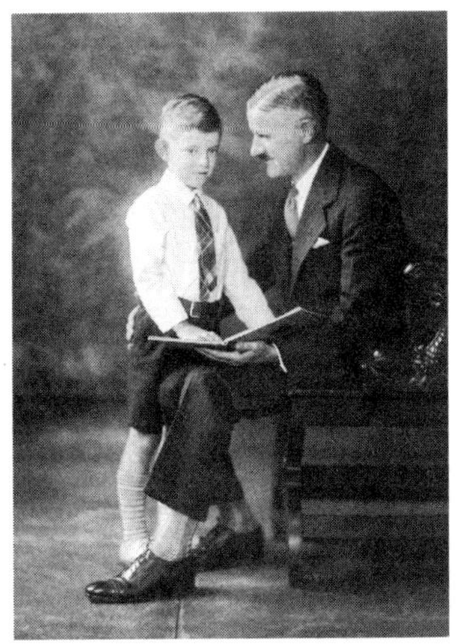

FIGURE 1.4. Mac and young Jack, age 8, 1928.

It took the determination of the wife of US Senator Millard E. Tydings of

Maryland to get the initiative started. A volunteer nurse's aid at Garfield, Eleanor Tydings, like many wives of politicians in Washington, demonstrated her patriotism during World War II by volunteering in the District's busy public hospitals. She was well connected to those in power and was outspoken when it came to reforming the aging and outdated hospitals she discovered.

One day while volunteering at Garfield, Eleanor Tydings was greeted by the sight of a rat scurrying across the hospital's main corridor.[13] At home she demanded immediate congressional attention to the deplorable hospital conditions, and her husband listened. Working with both Tydingses, Mac, now chief of surgery at Garfield and a strong voice in the DC medical society, finally had the political leverage he needed to move the aging public hospitals of Washington into the twentieth century.

The result of this work was the Washington Hospital Center Act, introduced in the US Senate in 1944 by Senator Tydings.[14] Tydings, a veteran of World War I, was well known for taking principled and sometimes controversial stands on various issues. A decade earlier, in 1934, he had offered a resolution to force President Roosevelt to publicly call Hitler to task for "discriminations and oppressions imposed by the Reich upon its Jewish citizens."[15] Although to his disappointment his foresight was bottlenecked by the Senate Foreign Relations Committee, Tydings remained a voice ahead of his time. He proved more successful in guiding the country's recognition of the Philippines as a separate and self-governing nation (Tydings-McDuffie Act)[16] and in reforming hospitals in the capital.

Despite his failing health, Mac worked tirelessly with Senator Tydings through the long and difficult political process that eventually culminated in President Harry Truman's signing the Washington Hospital Center Act on August 8, 1946. A personal note of appreciation to Mac from Eleanor Tydings celebrated the victory and applauded Mac's part in it:

> *July 31, 1946*
> *Dear Dr. McGovern,*
>
> *You must be as happy as I am over the passage of the DC Hospital Center Bill by the House of Representatives! It was a long, hard fight, culminating in a real battle on the floor of the House of Representatives, but we finally won out. Your testimony before the House Committee was one of the most effective blows struck on behalf of the Bill and I will never forget that crucial moment when you spoke to those men. . . . Your remarks were a powerful argument*

and had great effect. . . . My husband is at present in route home from the Philippines or he would join me in many thanks to you for your contribution to the passage of the Hospital Bill and warm regards and best wishes.
Sincerely Your Friend,
Eleanor D. Tydings[17]

Mac did not live to see the new Washington Hospital Center open its doors on March 10, 1958. It was one of the first hospitals in the area to have a tissue and eye bank, and one of the first in the country to be fully air-conditioned and to have computerized accounting systems and state-of-the art research laboratories.

Jack McGovern would always remember the conditions his father worked in through the Depression and the war years of the 1940s. And he would remember from Mac's example that a hard-working physician could have a significant impact on the bigger picture of health-care delivery and could better the prospects for his profession as well as for his patients. He had learned something lasting about service to the profession and about the focus and personal dedication required to be a catalyst for change.

Mac also served the military, as a member of the Medical Advisory Council of the National Selective Service System. In January 1941, nearly a year before the Japanese attack on Pearl Harbor, he was named chairman of the local procurement and assignment service for doctors in the War Manpower Commission. Local newspapers featured him as "Washingtonian of the Week." The *Washington Post* noted that the previous week Mac had "revealed that some 400 Washington physicians under the age of 45 are soon to receive written invitations to appear for an interview regarding military service. These are the men—the Army isn't taking lady doctors yet—whom Dr. McGovern's board has found to be available, after discussing their duties with the hospitals, medical schools and other institutions with which they are in association."[18] In this role Mac was instrumental in overseeing the selection of medical officers to serve their country during the busy war years of the early 1940s.

On May 6, 1942, the DC Medical Society presented Mac with a Certificate for Meritorious Service in recognition of his extraordinary contributions.[19] Jack McGovern would remember for a lifetime the pride he felt in his father's recognition by his peers. He came to see service as a necessary rather than an optional virtue, something to be practiced as a daily habit.

Just a year after being promoted to Chief of Surgery at Garfield Hospital, Mac McGovern was diagnosed with tuberculosis. That same year, 1945, he retired from his life in medicine just as his son graduated from medical school and began his own medical career. Mac's hope of overcoming his failing health and returning to the surgical practice he loved was not to be fulfilled. He died in 1951 at the young age of fifty-seven. Theodore Wiprud, a colleague at the DC medical society, penned a memorial to his friend:

> For four turbulent years he was Chairman of the Society's Executive Board. Although often hard-pressed, he never complained. Constitutionally he could not do things by halves and when the welfare of his medical organization was threatened, he gave everything he had without regard to the consequences to himself. If anyone served his fellow physicians "beyond the call of duty," he did. . . . A high sense of duty, common sense, unquestioned honesty, tolerance, friendliness, sympathy and good nature were his dominant characteristics. The welfare of his patients was always uppermost in his mind and that extended to his financial relationship with them.[20]

It was a tribute that Jack treasured.

Jack's mother, Lottie Brown McGovern, slender, pretty, and efficient, was a source of calm and comfort in her household. She had learned a superior domesticity from her mother and put it to good use. She could make a house attractive on a shoestring, and she took great pleasure in cookery and was renowned as a practitioner of that art. Thanksgiving and Christmas in Lottie's kitchen were fragrant with roasted turkey and its accompaniments; her cookies and pies were by all accounts unsurpassed. Often Lottie's married sister would assist her with special meals and celebrations. (Margaret, or "Aunt Sis," was a favorite of Jack's throughout his life, and his letters home in later years typically included the affectionate closing, "Please give my love to Aunt Sis.") Jack's roommate at Duke, Ziggy McPherson, later wrote that he had become "well acquainted" with Mac and Lottie. He described Mac as "a respected surgeon and teacher . . . a warm and gracious gentleman whom a person could readily admire." Lottie he described as "sweet and kind and an excellent cook, as demonstrated at Thanksgiving. She also would send us Jack's favorite macaroons."[21]

Years later McGovern, now an established physician of considerable wealth, would remind his aging, widowed mother, as she moved into a new apartment off Connecticut Avenue, how much he admired her domestic and managerial skills. She was meticulous and precise in her planning and had a close eye for detail.

> *October 5, 1964*
> *Dear Mother:*
> *I hope that your apartment is not too much of a mess since they painted it. I'll bet that it looks beautiful after you get it straightened out. You always have had a wonderful ability to make things look beautiful with a minimum amount of funds—I recall that our apartment always looked nice, even during the depression, and most of the rest of the time when we had very little money. You certainly are a wonderful manager! Please give my love to Aunt Sis and my best regards to all our friends in Washington.*
> *Love,*
> *Jack.*[22]

It will become clear in the pages to follow that both Jack's parents had tremendous influence on his developmental years, but his extended family and its roots in Irish culture were important, too. Jack's grandparents and their parents and their stories also contributed in many important ways to the man John McGovern would become.

Black Potatoes and Irishmen

Andrea Barrett's beautifully written *Ship Fever* provides a richly descriptive and representative portrait of the extraordinary pain and suffering experienced by the Irish during the Irish Potato Famine. Beginning in 1845 and for six long years thereafter, more than a million men, women, and children died in Ireland from starvation and disease caused by the failure of the annual potato crop. Barrett cites this letter by an anonymous Irishman traveling across the country with relief workers two years into the famine. It describes horrors he had seen with his own eyes, horrors carved deeply into the Irish psyche:

> At Arranmore in County Donegal, the streets swarm with famished men begging for work on the roads. At Louisburgh, in County Mayo, the local newspaper reports between ten and twenty deaths a day, and I myself saw

> bodies lying unburied, for want of anyone to dig a grave. In a hut that had been quiet for many days we found on the mud floor four frozen corpses, partly eaten by rats. That same day, a dispensary doctor told me he'd seen a woman drag from her hovel the corpse of her naked daughter. She tried to cover the body with stones.
>
> Does this give you some idea? Here at Skibbereen, I saw in one cabin a man, his wife, and two of their children, all emaciated beyond belief, sitting around a tiny fire and mourning a young child dead in her cradle, for whom they had no way to provide a coffin.[23]

McGovern's grandfather Philip provided young Jack his middle name and a background of grim Irish stories. The narrative of Irish anguish that was handed down to him by his family became part of Jack's mental landscape, too.

Of the Irish who survived the famine, an estimated two million, including many McGoverns, fled their homeland and emigrated to the United States, Canada, and Great Britain.[24] Eighty percent of the immigrants were Catholic.[25] Most of them lived in great poverty, few could read or write, and many suffered great hardships or even died in making their journey from their homeland. For all, it must have been unimaginably hard to leave a place they loved and risk everything in a foreign land. Three out of every four Irish emigrants settled in the United States with devastating memories of their homeland and the tragic events they had never seen coming.[26]

The potato crop planted in the summer of 1845 had appeared to be one of the best of the decade. Tiny purple flowers accented by large flat leaves and sturdy potato stalks could be seen for miles across the rolling Irish countryside. No one could predict the disappointment and deadly consequences fall would bring.

Most of Ireland's rural population—more than six million people—depended on these potatoes to feed their families through the year. More than two million acres had been sown, and from August to May the Irish would eat potatoes in every way imaginable—they boiled and roasted them and mashed them with buttermilk and onions. Their soup would be potato, their bread—potato.[27] In fact, some three million Irish peasants subsisted *solely* on the potato, which is rich in carbohydrates, minerals, and vitamins, including riboflavin, niacin, and Vitamin C. Irish peasants were actually healthier than peasants in Europe or England where bread, far less nutritious, was the staple food.

Potatoes in Ireland are harvested twice each fall, with new potatoes harvested in late August and the general crop of older potatoes, in October. But in the fall of 1845 things would be very different. There would be no potatoes. The culprit in the crisis was an airborne fungus, *Phytophthora infestans*, originally transported in the holds of ships traveling from North America to England. Potatoes that looked normal when pulled from the ground turned to black mush within days. Not only was there no food. Worse yet, there were no seeds for the next year's planting.

One of the most beautiful countries on the planet had descended into nightmare. And the memories of those who survived would furnish the imaginations of their descendants. John McGovern's paternal grandparents, Philip and Ann McGovern, born shortly after the famine, were among the many who never shook off their families' memories of those terrible times when the Irish left everything behind and sailed to America. Philip and Ann went to New York City before eventually settling in Washington, DC,[28] where they passed their stories down to a young Jack McGovern who no doubt listened wide-eyed to the tales of that very hot Irish summer in 1845 when the potatoes turned black.

The youngest McGovern heard these family tales and never let them go, although thanks to his grandparents' migration he himself had been born in the heart of the richest nation's capital, right in the middle of a gilded-age bubble that shimmered brightly in his world until it popped on October 29, 1929, with the stock market crash known as Black Tuesday. McGovern was then eight years old, and the stories in his head about the Irish Potato Famine became conflated with the awful economic collapse of unparalleled proportion that would persist into his high school years in the mid-1930s.

For a generation of young people, especially those born into the promising decade of the Roaring Twenties, when the good life was supposed only to get better, two lessons were conveyed by that ominous teacher the Great Depression: life is precious and easy to lose; money is hard to earn and easier to lose. Those lessons would not be lost on Jack McGovern. Other lessons would come from more genial teachers—his maternal grandparents and extended family.

Granny Brown and the Extended Family

As much as Jack McGovern loved his mother and her sister, Aunt Sis, his maternal grandmother, Granny Brown, held a very special place in his heart. Mary Fahrnkoff Brown was pure German in heritage. Her father, John Fahrnkoff, had come from Germany in 1853, arriving in New York City on June 24 at the age of thirty-eight.[29] He soon settled in Washington, DC.

Mary would become the wife of George Brown, one of six brothers, the sons of Charlotte Ann Brown and James Lemuel Brown. Another of the six brothers was Francis Brown, who becomes important to this story because he married a Hayes, Essie Hayes, and their only child would be Jack McGovern's famous second cousin, the Academy Award-winning actress Helen Hayes. The Browns' ancestry was English, and the Browns were especially proud of that fact, for they had come to the United States before the American Revolution and considered their lineage much better than that of poor Irish immigrants such as the McGoverns and the Hayeses.

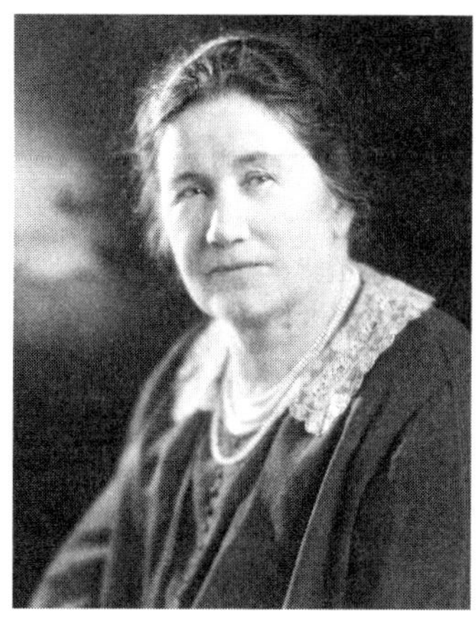

FIGURE 1.5. Mary Fahrnkoff Brown, Jack McGovern's beloved Granny Brown.

Granny Brown had a broad, handsome, congenial face and comfortable ways. She was Jack's great favorite and a central figure during his formative years. She and his grandfather Brown lived in a farmhouse outside the city. That beautiful two-story house with its covered porch and chickens scratching in the front yard no longer exists. What was then a country farm surrounded by fields and forest is now a busy suburban parking lot off Georgia Avenue.

In those days at the Brown farm there were horses and barnyard fowl, broad open spaces, and ponds in which to fish. Indoors, Granny held forth in her kitchen—which had been the original training school for Lottie's acclaimed culinary skills. But Granny Brown endeared herself to her grandson not only through her cookery but also through her generosity of heart and her willingness to help people in need. Jack recalled seeing her basement opened up often as a makeshift dining room for hungry people in search of a hot meal during the Depression.[30]

Hardly a weekend went by that Jack was not at Granny Brown's. From the McGoverns' apartment and later their house near Connecticut Avenue, he could make the journey by city bus across Rock Creek Park and north up Georgia Avenue in good time. There in the country he had a second home, and one where, on a very good day, Brother Frank would drop in and take him fishing.

Granny Brown was the family matriarch—an authority figure who gave her grandson advice about life that he could literally take to the bank. In his own words:

> I must have been about seven or eight and I had managed to save some money from my paper route. I was also a stamp collector and helped a gentleman in our apartments sell stamps by approval to a list of clients who would receive books of US postal stamps in the mail for their collections. They would select from the book the stamps they wanted, send in a payment, and then mail the book of stamps (less those they purchased) to the next person on the list. In time, I would get the picked over books and we would refill them with more stamps to make another round. In this way I got paid a few cents per mailing and between paper route and stamps I managed to save up $7 dollars—my first $7 dollars.
>
> I asked my grandmother what I should do with such a large amount of money and she said give it to a bank. I couldn't understand why I would give my hard earned money to a bank but she explained they would pay me interest. I had to ask what in the heck interest was and then she explained they would keep my money safe and pay me more for keeping it. Well, I thought that sounded like a pretty good idea after I confirmed a couple of times that I could get all my money back when I needed it, including interest.[31]

Grandmother Brown's advice was well placed. In the mind of young Jack, if a few dollars could make money for him by doing nothing but sitting in a bank, then a few hundred dollars, a few thousand dollars . . . well, the possibilities were endless.

That well-worn bank deposit book from the Perpetual Building Association, 11th and E Street NW, Washington, DC, exists to this day with Jack's name proudly scripted at the top over his mother's signature as parent/guardian. Its first line records a seven-dollar deposit on May 27, 1929, and shows the first dividend paid by the bank, on July 1, 1929, in the amount of ten cents.[32] Fortunately many banks in Washington fared better during the Depression than others in the country, and Jack's first deposit was not lost. From this meager deposit of seven dollars, an investment career and a future foundation were launched.

Jack was a frequent correspondent with his maternal grandparents. He provided them with timely reports of his many activities during his teens, including summer camps, Boy Scouts, sandlot baseball, and studies at school. One letter arrived from summer vacation just a week after his first savings account was established. The interest from savings earned by selling stamps was obviously on his mind. The spelling is his.

> *July 12, 1929*
>
> *Dear granmother we arrived at sherwood forest all right. I am going to join the scouts. I think I will have lots of fun. I like it down here fine. I went for a long walk yesterday. How is grandpa getting along? Mother and Aunt Sis are having a nice time. Keep the stamps over at your house and save the stamp on this letter.—Jack*[33]

Throughout high school McGovern would build his stamp collection. More than just stamps, his collection was a window on the world, one that contributed its mite to a lifelong love of history. He liked knowing the stories behind the famous faces and institutions his stamps commemorated. Jack was a collector at heart, and every collection was an investment with value and could be sold or traded for something of greater value. In time he would sell his collection of stamps to help cover some expenses of an education that would provide him enough income to generate the larger collections of rare medical books and investment portfolios that would shape his legacy.

Cousin Helen

Helen Hayes has been called the first lady of the American theater for good reason. Born October 10, 1900, to Francis Brown and his Irish wife, Catherine Estelle Hayes, or Essie, Helen would follow her mother's dreams onto the stage at the tender age of five. As a child star and as an adult, she conquered stage and screen and became one of America's great treasures—a woman who could claim Oscar, Grammy, Emmy, and Tony awards along with the Presidential Medal of Freedom.

Proud as he was of his older cousin, to Jack she was simply a cousin. After all, her father, Francis Van Arnum Brown, was his maternal grandfather's brother. Late in his life, during his seventh decade, McGovern dictated some recollections about her and her branch of the family:

> Helen's father's education would have been limited to no more than high school. His Brown ancestry came from England but I have heard from my mother that there was some touch of Welsh. My great grandmother Brown, mother of Francis Van Arnum, felt that Francis had married beneath them; that the bride's family were poor Irish immigrants. . . . My mother often told me of the kind gentleman that was her Grandfather Francis Brown.
>
> On a personal note, I clearly heard from my mother that Helen's mother, and to a considerable degree Helen, did not think highly of Francis. Francis lived 'retired' from being a successful salesman and lived alone in a cottage in Sherwood Forest, apparently doing nothing. They both thought that he should be doing something productive. I only met him once as a young child at his cabin and thought that he was friendly and funny, in a good sense.
>
> My grandfather, George Brown, was the oldest of the brothers and had retired in Washington many years before I was born and we often visited him and my grandmother, who was a most wonderful person of German ancestry on both sides. . . . I first met Helen Hayes when she came over to visit her Uncle George but really, I think, loved my Grandmother even more as did most everybody. I was about seven years old when I met her at Grandmother's—I had been told that she was a famous actress. Needless to say, I was really impressed when she drove up in a bright yellow car with the roof down. When she came up the steps and I was there with Granddad on the porch, the first thing she wanted was to talk to me, noting she had heard so much about her cousin, Jack.[34]

From the day Helen Hayes stepped out of that yellow convertible in his grandmother's yard, she was Jack McGovern's role model for what one person could accomplish through focus, hard work, practiced talent, and a bit of calculated risk.

Helen's grandfather Patrick Hayes had also immigrated to the Washington, DC, area from Ireland shortly after the potato famine. He was the nephew of Catherine Hayes, known as the Swan of Erin, a singer beloved throughout Ireland, who became the toast of London as well when she performed at the Royal Albert Hall.[35] Patrick also had the gift of a fine voice, but the story goes that he had been struck in the eye by a piece of flint and eventually lost his vision and his job, and found refuge in the bottle.

Patrick was a devout Catholic whose religious zeal so tormented the people around him that, Helen recalled, the rest of the family would in time become "very easy" in their faith.[36] Patrick's wife, Graddy, was of English descent; together they had two daughters and a son, the eldest being Essie, Helen's mother. In Helen's words:

> I should love to have known my father Francis Van Arnum Brown before he grew up to be my father. But then—he never did grow up really. He never deserted his boyhood but remained content with the tiniest successes. Mother chose the least aggressive of the five Brown brothers as her own. He married for love of the spirited and witty Irish girl, against his mother's wishes. . . . He married for love and a home; she married for escape from home. He wanted peace; she wanted freedom. The young Browns were at odds from the start, and when I came along I only made matters worse.[37]

Helen's mother would live vicariously through her daughter's success onstage and in movies. The two would be on the road for months at a time, leaving Helen's father behind. Young Jack greatly admired his older cousin for her success and national acclaim. Through Helen he could envision the good life and the opportunities that hard work in a chosen career could provide when coupled with careful investments—something he was just learning about.

Helen married a successful young Chicago journalist and playwright, a life-of-the-party sort named Charlie MacArthur. Their adopted son, James MacArthur, would become a successful actor and the co-star of the well-known television series *Hawaii Five-O,* which ran twelve seasons, from 1968 to 1980. Helen's daughter, Mary, followed her mother onto the stage, but, tragically, died of polio in 1949 at the age of nineteen. The loss was devastating to Helen and even more so to Charlie, who never seemed to get over it. He died in 1956, just four years after Mac McGovern. The determination with which Helen rose above her grief and continued her career with dignity and great success was a source of pride to her younger cousin Jack, whose own struggle was with the death of his father.

From Helen's autobiography, *On Reflection,* we get a rare snapshot of what the Hayes, Brown, and McGovern extended family life was like in Washington during young Jack's adolescence when the whole clan would gather for Christmas:

> I remember sprawling, apple-cheeked children and chattering women with aprons, bustling in cozy, cooking-sweet rooms, tending their men folk. . . . It all seemed like one long holiday. The faintest whiff of pine or peppermint and I am carried back to the most wonderful times of all, those first and best Christmases. Preparations would start in November. Father and I and the Brown cousins and the Hayeses, too, would all go into the woods to hunt black walnuts, and we must sometimes have invaded private property because I recall being chased by cows. Then we would all run for cover.

When plans for Christmas began, Helen recorded, the children went to work:

> We were now given reams of paper, scissors, and pots of homemade paste. Our job was to make the traditional colored-paper chains for decorations. Then there was popcorn-stringing and after that was over, we all settled down—Sissie and Lottie Brown and George and all the cousins—to make our gifts: terrible tie racks with Indian heads and cedar boxes with awful designs. My poor uncles and aunts! . . . even the good gifts, given to us by the grownups, were homemade. These were usually beautiful, though the materials never cost more than a dollar and a half. Anyway, by the time the tree was dressed, the apples hung on branches to weigh them, the boxes placed at its base, it was really Christmas—and the like of it will not come again.[38]

Another annual ritual for Jack was baseball and the Washington Senators. Jack's love of the game was intensified by his father's fame as a college all-star; this was "semi-pro" status, according to his proud son. His love of the game can also be traced to his grandfather George and to Helen's father, Francis, these brothers being compulsive fans who rarely missed a game of their hometown Washington Senators. To live in Washington in the early 1900s was to spend Sundays rooting for the Senators and Walter Johnson, "the greatest pitcher ever to walk on the field," according to the Brown brothers.[39]

Cotton candy, hotdogs, baseball at Griffith Stadium, John Philip Sousa conducting red, white, and blue marches at the bandstand next to the Washington Monument, the Glen Echo Amusement Park with its famous Ferris wheel—these all made glorious childhood memories that Helen and Jack would share over the years.[40]

Griffith Stadium was especially wonderful. Named after the Washington Senators' manager and owner, Clark Griffith, it was a place where a schoolboy could watch the president throw out the first ball of the season (every president from Harding to JFK would follow the tradition) and see history being made as the likes of Babe Ruth rounded the bases. The old scoreboard was shaped like a beer bottle and towered nearly fifty feet into the air and was operated manually. Some skill and much attention to the game were required to flip the numbers as runners crossed home plate. One young man who was especially attentive at running the scoreboard would one day grow up to be the Commissioner of Major League Baseball—his name, Bowie Kuhn.[41]

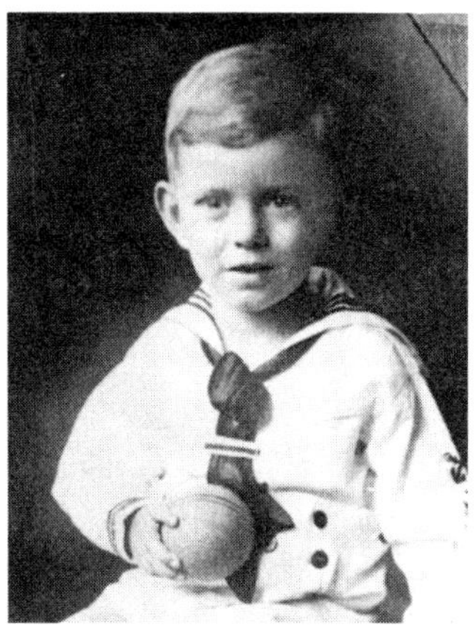

FIGURE 1.6. Jack at about five.

Games were played in the daytime; outdoor light to illuminate the field after dark did not appear until the 1940s. Although the Washington team had some less than stellar years (immortalized in the Broadway musical *Damn Yankees*), their fortunes seemed to change in 1920, the season before Jack was born, thus providing him something his elders never had—a winning team led by Hall-of-Famers, including Bucky Harris, Goose Goslin, Sam Rice, and the seemingly ageless Walter Johnson. And throughout his childhood Jack watched and marveled at the accomplishments of Babe Ruth, who sent thrills through the whole country. Ruth retired from baseball in 1935, just as the Jack entered Woodrow Wilson High School.

As his own medical and investment careers commanded notice on a national scale in the 1960s and 1970s, Jack would grow closer to Helen. Her philanthropy in the arts provided additional inspiration for him. She was seriously afflicted by allergies, said to be linked to her years working around dusty stages, and as a result attended Jack's Houston allergy clinic annually, where she credited her now prosperous cousin with saving her career. She would die of congestive heart failure March 17, 1993, at the age of ninety-two at her home in Nyack, New York. It was St. Patrick's day—a fitting day for the last exit of the Irish first lady of the American theater.

Recalled McGovern in a note dictated after Helen's death: "[Over the years] we had intermitting visits . . . we would visit with her in Cuernavaca, Mexico and many times at her home in Nyack, New York. She visited us . . . at our winter home in Palm Desert a number of times but often in Houston where she came to be treated in our clinic for her allergies. We became very close and she also truly loved my wife."[42]

At seventy-nine, Helen wrote a quick note to be included in the appreciations book celebrating McGovern's thirty-five years in medicine:

> Once I had a young cousin, a lad with blond hair and ears a little outstanding and blinking, light blue eyes, and a great shyness.
>
> He also had a great dedication, the latter has led that shy lad to become one of the most distinguished doctors in America and the pride of the family of which I am a grateful member.
>
> That is Dr. John P. McGovern, my cousin, Jack, who not only has given me great happiness shining in his reflected glory, but also has lengthened my life by his uncanny spotting of the one great weakness in my otherwise iron constitution. He has conquered my allergy and given me a whole new life.
>
> I am grateful to the doctor and proud of the cousin and loving of the man. And, oh yes, he has become quite handsome in his maturity.[43]

DC Public Schools

In the early 1920s, Washington, DC, was overhauling its public school system to make the District a model for public education. For years the segregated public schools of the District had been deteriorating in quality and public perception. The conclusion of World War I signaled a new opportunity to improve them to meet the needs of the District's growing suburbs like Cleveland Park and Tenleytown, where so many young

Washingtonians like the McGoverns were starting their families and recognizing that the key to their children's future would be education. The suburb of Cleveland Park had evolved from a thousand-acre farm belonging to General Uriah Forrest, aide-de-camp to George Washington. The community, just four miles from the White House, is built in the area of Fort Reno, one of the largest of the forts that provided a protective barrier around Washington during the Civil War. At 429 feet above sea level, it has the distinction of being the highest natural point in the district.

These suburbs grew rapidly as the advent of Henry Ford's mass-produced Model T, affectionately known as the Tin Lizzy, took the nation by storm during Jack's childhood. Fewer than a half million motorcars existed in 1910. But during the next decade they became a necessity for Americans. Two years before Jack's birth in 1921 there were seven million cars in the country. By his eighth birthday in 1929—23 million.[44]

The expansion of the Washington suburbs precipitated a community outcry for more services outside the District's core. High on the list was the demand for sweeping improvements to the public schools. From 1847 forward, citizens in the District of Columbia had had little to say about their school policies and even less about budget issues. Acts of 1874 and 1878 forbade bond issues, and all public projects since had been pay-as-you-go, with Congress fixing every budgetary detail.[45] By 1900 the board of education had won the right to choose the superintendent and the assistant superintendents—one for the white schools and one for the black, since the schools were, in keeping with the times, racially segregated. In 1906 a new law vested in the judges of the District's supreme court the appointment of the board's nine members—six white and three black.

One would think that, being located just miles from the headquarters of the nation's seat of education (including the Office of Education, the National Education Association, and the American Council on Education), the DC school district would be at the top of its game regarding curricula, teaching methodology, and facilities. But that simply was not the case. World War I had a curious effect on DC schools. The public schools for blacks actually gained ground on the white schools. Both suffered from congressional disregard resulting from the war efforts ongoing at the time. But the war generated higher-paying jobs outside the schools, which many of the best white teachers could not resist, thus creating a brain drain in the white schools. While the segregated black schools had outstanding teachers of their own, these, for the most part, stayed with their schools. The hiring practices of the era made it harder for them to move into the newly opened jobs. At the same time, between 1917 and 1919 the white schools saw an increase of enrollment to more than 44,300 students, but had a schoolroom capacity of only 36,000.[46]

During the fall of 1921, when Lottie Brown McGovern was pregnant with her son, a comprehensive reorganization of the DC public schools was underway. The citizens of neighborhoods like Tenleytown and Cleveland Park demanded more of their schools and were up in arms over their deteriorating condition and thin curriculum. The superintendent of schools had to go. In his place, a well-respected assistant superintendent of Boston Schools, Frank W. Ballou, was recruited. Ballou was more than up to the task and took on all the issues, including the financial problems, the congressional committees still loyal to the former superintendent, and the immediate need to build a new working relationship with the black schools.[47]

With a PhD in education from Harvard University, experience acquired in Cincinnati and Boston, and a bulldog personality backed by unabashed self-confidence, Ballou took on every challenge and succeeded. He remained superintendent for more than two decades and during that time turned a dilapidated public school system into one of the best systems in the nation.

For starters, he spent a year collecting data and compiling a comprehensive report, which he presented to the Board of Education in 1922 under the title "Why Educational Progress in Washington Is So Slow." "Education conditions in Washington," the report boldly stated, "are among the worst to be found in any city in the Union." It added, "Until Congress can be made to realize that it is incompetent properly to administer such an undertaking and will give the Board of Education the power and control which should belong to it there is little hope of a good, modern school system for the District of Columbia."[48] Ballou's report went on to provide solutions and recommendations that would turn the tide and reverse the course of DC's schools in the near future.

All of this, of course, worked to the advantage of the newest McGovern in North Cleveland Park. He and hundreds of Washington newborns in 1921 would in a few years be attending new elementary, junior high, and high schools that Superintendent Ballou launched—each supported by higher-paid teachers, new curricula, and a spirit of innovation. The gods of formative education were shining on John P. McGovern.

McGovern's primary school, Ben W. Murch Elementary, was erected in 1929 on the site of the phased-out Grant Road School that dated back to the 1870s, when Congress had first established a public school system for the District.[49] The new Ben W. Murch Elementary was a modern, well-staffed school that provided an outstanding start to its students—and was right around the corner from the McGoverns' apartment on Connecticut Avenue.

The location of Mac and Lottie's apartment, and of the house to follow in the same neighborhood, assured Jack a smooth transition through his entire public school education. What were now considered some of the best public schools the nation had to offer were all within walking distance of the McGovern home.

Jack's junior high school, Alice Deal Junior High, was completed in 1931 on land acquired from the Fort Reno site. Construction began in August 1930, and the school opened on September 23, 1931. The school's namesake, Alice Deal (1877–1928), was a math teacher at McKinley Manual Training School and the founder of Washington's junior high school system.[50] The school was very active both academically and socially, and of special interest is the fact that it focused on science. There was an excellent science lab where the students performed experiments, made terrariums, and were exposed to biological sciences at a level not provided in former schools. Records reveal that "Heel and Tie" day was the big event of the month. On that day the girls would wear stockings and high heels and the boys would wear suits and ties, and there would be dancing in the gym with a live band in the afternoon.[51]

With the addition of a new elementary and junior high school, the community, led by the Forest Hills Citizens Association, pushed for a new high school to be built on the Fort Reno grounds near Alice Deal Junior High. At the time, high school students from the area were sent to Western High School, which was rapidly becoming overcrowded. In fact, the association suggested that the entire Reno section should be bought up for a school, parks, and recreational purposes. In February 1931 Congress granted an appropriation of $180,000 to purchase the site. By December 1931, 6.5 acres had been bought for $109,700 to build the high school, which would open September 3, 1935. It opened three months ahead of schedule.[52]

Sitting high on the hill adjacent to the original Fort Reno, the new school, Woodrow Wilson High, struck a handsome profile and was the talk of the town. The new brick edifice housed a gym, ample classrooms, well-trained teachers, and one of the fanciest home economics facilities in the city, complete with a cooking lab. Another innovative feature was the courtyard off the armory, where the cadets would drill. A large auditorium was soon added.

The new high school sponsored a wide variety of clubs, and belonging to one was important to almost every student. There were clubs for riding, badminton, drama, hockey, tennis, and various languages. There was a swim team that practiced at the YMCA. Y-Teens was a very popular club that raised money and gave parties for underprivileged children in the community.

Jack McGovern, outgoing as he was, took advantage of the many opportunities. His high school yearbook notes that he was a member of the Chevrons Club (which was a Cadet Corps), the Panel Club (which organized panel discussions on timely topics), the Cadet Band (in which he was a corporal), and the honor and debate societies.[53] Although he was recognized for his talent at playing baseball throughout his childhood and in junior high, Jack struggled to make the freshman squad in high school due to his small size. He would forever be lean and small-framed; in adulthood, he was five feet, eight inches tall. Recognizing that his size would always limit a standout career in sports, he switched his focus to his other great interest, medicine.[54]

Jack's high school yearbook provides an interesting snapshot of the times. His classmates voted *You Can't Take It With You* as best movie of the year; Charlie McCarthy as favorite radio star; Spencer Tracy and Hedy Lamarr as favorite movie stars; and Artie Shaw as most popular orchestra, almost a tie with Tommy Dorsey.[55]

While the McGovern family lived in apartments off Connecticut Avenue during Jack's elementary schooling and his first two years of junior high, in the mid-1930s both father and mother had their eye on single-family dwellings being built a block west of Connecticut Avenue. The homes were just a short walk or bicycle ride up the steep hill to the city's newest and best public schools. When their son was fourteen, in 1935, Mac and Lottie bought a comfortable new two-story brick home at 3601 Cumberland Street. It had a handsome fireplace, four bedrooms, three baths, a basement, an attached garage, and a fenced backyard. The new house was around the corner from the family's apartment building and a block closer to the schools up the hill at Reno Park. Here the McGoverns would establish themselves in a neighborhood of upward-moving middle-class Washingtonians—a neighborhood that exists today with little change, known now as it was then for good location, good schools, and family-friendliness.

The purchase of a home just blocks away from the apartments and busy traffic of Connecticut Boulevard perhaps signaled a family celebration of sorts, given that the worst years of the Great Depression were now behind them. Mac's growing son and increasing recognition as a respected surgeon at Garfield and a leader in the DC medical society required more than the small apartment that had hitherto served the family so well.

Jack, now a teenager, lived in a home at the foot of Reno Park, where Alice Deal Junior High and Woodrow Wilson High towered over the community—a community whose past concerns about invading Confederate soldiers were now replaced with current concerns that their children have access to a first-rate education. The DC public schools would provide a golden ticket to the best colleges and to the "American Dream", a

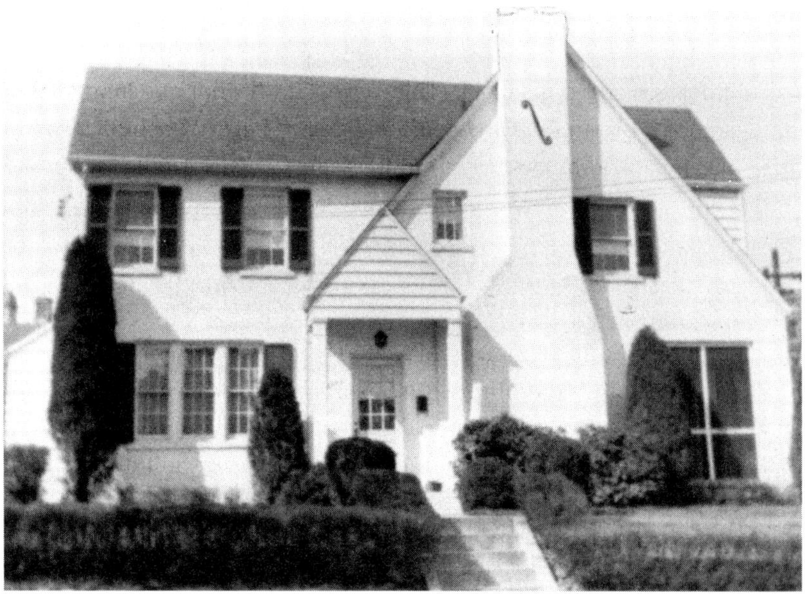

FIGURE 1.7. McGovern's childhood home at 3601 Cumberland Street, as it looked in 1936.

term newly coined by historian James Truslow Adams in his 1931 classic, *The Epic of America*.[56]

Today the home at 3601 Cumberland Street is well preserved and as charming as it must have been when the McGoverns lived there. It is easy to look at the house now and to imagine another day, when a young Jack McGovern flew around the corner on his bike headed up the hill to Alice Deal Junior High.

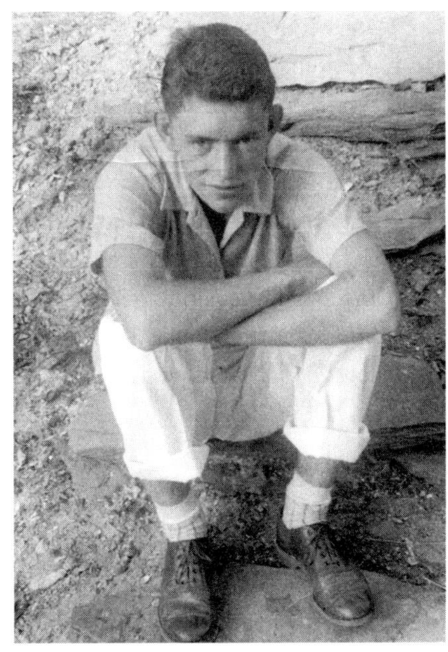

FIGURE 1.8. Jack McGovern as a teenager.

Playing for all the Marbles

Step forward in time.

"Have you ever played marbles?" an elderly Jack McGovern asked me one night as we sat in his apartment overlooking the Texas Medical Center. I replied that, well, yes, I more or less remembered shooting a few marbles with the kids in my neighborhood a time or two, but that I wasn't very good at it.

"No, no," McGovern said, dismissing half-hearted, half-remembered marbles. "I'm talking about a *real* game of marbles—ringer. A ten-foot circle with thirteen marbles in a cross at its center. I'm talking lag lines, pitch lines, and knuckling down to knock the most marbles at center from the ring."

No, I hadn't played that kind of marbles.

Then he acknowledged his humble beginnings in the marble stakes. He had started out with a bunch of cheap glass marbles and by dint of long practice had become very good at the game. He had set his eye on the prize—agates. Agates were the best of marbles; they had great value, whereas glass marbles had very little. And he soon realized that if he put a whole jar of cheap, scratched glass marbles up against one or two agates, boys for blocks around could not resist the temptation; they would cheerfully put their good agates at risk for such an impressive quantity of junk.

At this point in his narrative McGovern looked up at the ceiling and proceeded to recreate an entire marble match that took place in 1930, from the first shot to the last. In his mind's eye he was nine years old again and "knuckling down" with his deadly accurate shooter, striking marble after marble from the ring. Not only did he walk away with most of his own cheap marbles; in less than a year, he notes with his wide grin, he owned most of the agates in Tinleytown.

I find this story of McGovern's interesting partly, of course, because it demonstrates his astonishing ability in his seventies to recall shot-by-shot a marble match from his youth. But it is interesting chiefly because it demonstrates facts critical to his immense success in accumulating money. One of these is that his drive to amass things of value (or beauty or use, to himself or other people) was unstoppable; it could not be deflected. He didn't just want *some* agates; he wanted *all* the agates, and the drive to get them imbued him with an unparalleled work ethic that made him practice his skills until they surpassed those of the people he was competing against. The combination of skill and drive was unbeatable; it enabled him to corner the agate market in the neighborhood. Furthermore, even at this marble-playing age McGovern understood the principle of leverage—he knew that he could use glass marbles to get agates and that owning the prize agates put him in a position to take on other goals he had in mind. The story of the marbles is an exemplar for McGovern's whole career.

The second part of this story also demonstrates a youthful Jack using a tactic that he would repeat throughout his life, specifically, taking advantage of the opportunity at hand. Jack wanted a bicycle, but his father refused to accede to his request for one. They lived near busy streets, and the danger was too great; he and Lottie would worry continuously. Mac was unrelenting, and repeated attempts to change his mind were unsuccessful.

Then one charmed day Jack spotted the perfect bicycle a block away. It belonged to a former agate owner. In spite of his father's impending disapproval, Jack traded some of his agates for the bike.

When his father came home from the hospital that evening, his displeasure at the sight of the bicycle was manifest. But before he could protest, Jack swung into an explanation of how he had come by it in a fair trade and already had a plan in place to assure his safety. His father listened; and the upshot of the conversation was a week's trial. During it, Jack succeeded in impressing his parents with his responsibility in matters concerning the preservation of life and limb, and the bicycle issue was laid to rest.

In addition to snatching an opportunity when it presented itself, Jack had on this occasion once more set a goal, kept his eyes on it, created leverage, and gotten what he wanted. And all of this had been made possible by the hours of practice that had supplied his stock of agates.[57] Playing for all the marbles is more than a story about McGovern's childhood; it is a motif reasserting itself throughout his lifetime of accomplishments in both medicine and business. His quest for agates of many shapes, from bicycles to clinics to investments, was a function of the competitive nature ingrained in his psyche from childhood.

Jack McGovern was not the only product of Washington, DC, who was fine-tuning his acquisition skills for the future. Another young man, eight years his junior, had moved into the community, and he also had a special talent for collecting and saving. His father was a newly elected member of Congress from Omaha, Nebraska. The son's name—Warren Buffett.

Buffett would follow in McGovern's footsteps, attending both Alice Deal Junior High and Woodrow Wilson High School.[58] Both boys' yearbooks would be prophetic enough to be interesting. McGovern's 1939 Tigers yearbook predicted that Jack would be remembered for his "broad grin, his natural business ability and broad philatelic knowledge, and his practical, aggressive character."[59] Next to Warren Buffett's senior picture in his 1947 Tigers yearbook would be the words "future stock broker."[60]

Medicine as a Vocation

One can only imagine the teenager who would become John P. McGovern, MD, racing up the street on his bike to Alice Deal Junior High with a meticulously bound research paper tucked tightly under his arm. It is his first research paper and he's out for an A. It may come as no surprise that the paper's title reads, "Medicine as a Vocation." The hand-typed, nine-page, double-spaced report bound with brass brads has its title carefully drawn in block letters above a drawing of an Erlenmeyer flask. Each page has been typed and retyped many times over, until there are no flaws to be found.

In this paper the reader is introduced to Hippocrates and the history of medicine, modern professional standards, and the young McGovern's interpretation of the requirements for the medical profession (which he explains include "a vigorous body," because "meals, sleep, and exercise will be irregular"). Essentials, he adds, also include a "cheerful temperament,

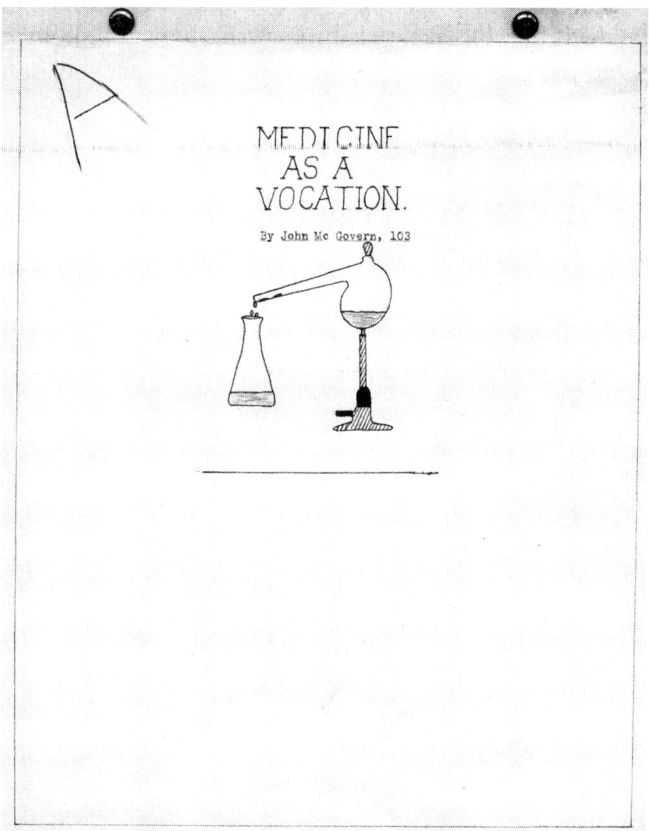
A

MEDICINE
AS A
VOCATION.

By John Mc Govern, 103

FIGURE 1.9. McGovern's first junior high school research paper.

optimistic nature, honesty of purpose, and love of work." He concludes with a comprehensive review of college requirements and a graph demonstrating the number of physicians and nurses who have graduated from US medical and nursing schools between 1880 and 1930.

It is obvious from the paper that at a very young age, Jack McGovern has set his eye on a lofty prize, a medical degree. In the words of the essay:

> The requirements for the physician are hard—mentally, physically, and financially—the profession demands from 7 to 10 of the best years of his life in intense study. We shall now see what rewards the physician receives for his labor.
>
> REWARDS—The physician gives much of his time to work done

> without remuneration for the alleviation of suffering among the poor. The motive that should prompt a young man to study medicine should be his desire to do something humane for his fellow man. If this is his motive, he trains himself well, and has a reasonably acceptable personality, his material reward will naturally come as his practice increases. The greatest reward the doctor has, however, is the knowledge and appreciation of the fact that he has accomplished something really beneficial to the welfare of humanity in general.
>
> The physician usually has no stated salary. Much of his financial success depends, of course, upon his location and professional ability; something depends too upon his business ability, high scientific attainments not always being combined with good business sense.[61]

This first junior high school research paper, meticulous and precise to the letter, provides a picture of the physician to be. His grade, as you might expect—A.

Off to College

In 1939 Jack's high school education was complete. His friends had urged him to go to Duke, but Drexel University in Philadelphia had also been a consideration. At just 136 miles from family and home, Drexel had a rich history dating back to 1848 and offered both undergraduate and medical school opportunities. But Duke was a contemporary university with a new medical school on the rise that could not be ignored. Several of McGovern's high school friends were going there, and the idea of being both farther from home and among friends must have been attractive.

The pull of Duke was strong. In fact, Duke was written in McGovern's stars, and it was on Duke that he settled, in the hills of Durham, North Carolina, where he would earn undergraduate and medical degrees over the next six years, 1939–1945.

Chapter Two

The Osler/Davison Connection

TO UNDERSTAND JOHN P. MCGOVERN is to know Wilburt Cornell Davison (1892–1972) and Sir William Osler (1849–1919). Davison, a Rhodes scholar, trained with Osler at Oxford during the years 1913–1916, then returned to the United States to complete a medical degree at Johns Hopkins and join the pediatrics faculty. In 1927 he was recruited from Baltimore to Durham as the founding dean of the Duke University School of Medicine. There he would build the school from the ground up, opening its doors in 1930. Nine years later Jack McGovern arrived at Duke for his undergraduate college years in hopes of being admitted to the medical school Davison had built.

The Osler/Davison/McGovern connection was a bond that helped shape McGovern's professional life. Osler influenced Davison in profound ways.[1] And Davison, in turn, influenced McGovern and the entire generation of young men and women who trained at the Duke University School of Medicine during the Davison years.[2] McGovern's respect for Davison and his gratitude to him burst out in a heartfelt encomium years later, in 1966, when he was forty-five years old, in a letter to the beloved mentor, whose "greatness," he wrote, " . . . has been my profoundest source of inspiration during these past 22 years." He went on:

> No one who has known you and basked in your sunshine can really ever be the same thereafter, for you have that magical quality that inspires men to grow. . . .

> Yours is a strong and wonderful phenomenon, difficult to define for us lesser men, for it must be compounded of indefinable qualities of heart and spirit and mind that are combined harmoniously only in the greatest of men. . . . No doubt Osler, and perhaps Welch, had certain of these qualities in good measure, and, from everything that I read about Osler and in contemplation of your own expressed feelings for him, he must have had. All that I can say is that I have never known or met anyone during my 45 years of existence who has whatever it is that I am talking about to the high degree embodied in yourself.[3]

At Dean Davison's memorial service held in the chapel at Duke on November 17, 1972, a clearly shaken McGovern turned to Shakespeare to express his loss: "And so I pay tribute to my lifelong hero and benefactor in medicine whose life so enriched my own that I can truly say about the Dean what Hamlet said about his father: 'He was a man, take him for all in all. I shall not look upon his like again.'"[4]

The Osler Connection

Who was the mentor's mentor?

Few who knew young Willie Osler as a boy growing up in Bond Head, Ontario, near Toronto, could imagine that the prankster who played practical jokes on them would one day become one of the most beloved and influential physicians of all time. After all, in 1866, when he was fourteen, Osler and his schoolmates barricaded the door of the school housekeeper and subjected her to the noxious fumes of molasses, pepper, and mustard heated on the schoolroom stove. For this he was expelled from school and sentenced to two days in jail, in addition to which he merited a mention the *Toronto Globe* in an article headed "School Row at Weston. Pupils Turned Outlaws. They Fumigate the Matron with Sulfur."[5]

Born in 1849 to an Anglican clergyman and his wife, William Osler began his undergraduate studies at Trinity College in Toronto with the intention of following his father's footsteps into the ministry. But his developing interest in the natural sciences, for which he was suited by a fine intellect and keen powers of observation, soon led him to medicine. The Reverend William Arthur Johnson and two physicians, James Bovell and Palmer Howard, were early mentors who nurtured his interests. Johnson and Bovell gave him access to his first microscope and medical books. Howard fueled his love for clinical care and teaching.

In 1868 Osler entered the Toronto Medical School; by 1870 he had moved to the McGill University School of Medicine in Montreal, which was considered to offer the best medical education in Canada. He graduated in 1872 and then, as was common at the time, set off to Europe with the object of seeing and learning from the best physicians and scientists of the day. In London, Berlin, and Vienna he furthered his education and built a broad foundation in physiology, medicine, pathology, surgery, neurology, and dermatology.

This added study made it possible for Osler to return to McGill to begin his teaching and clinical practice. He rose rapidly to the rank of professor. With funds from his own pocket he introduced the first course in clinical microscopy in Canada, and he cheerfully took charge of the smallpox wards and volunteered to perform autopsies—undertakings other faculty happily handed off to the energetic young man.

Osler's growing reputation as a teacher and pathologist/clinician led to his recruitment in 1884 as chair of clinical medicine at the University of Pennsylvania in Philadelphia. A beloved faculty member at McGill and a rising star in the profession, Osler agonized for days over leaving McGill and Canada before finally resorting to a coin toss. It came up heads, and Osler went to Pennsylvania.[6]

In Philadelphia Osler excelled as a professor of clinical medicine. His legend grew as he led his students into the wards for bedside instruction (novel at the time) and followed that up with regular hands-on teaching sessions in the Blockley deadhouse. Conducting more than a thousand autopsies, Osler developed an understanding of the natural history of disease that few others in medicine could match.

At One West Franklin Street, Osler started a tradition of providing latchkeys to his home for students and faculty so that they could use his growing library to continue their medical studies late into the night. He rejoiced at showing off a new medical book while sharing his love of medical history. His reputation as the outstanding teacher and clinician of his day grew rapidly during his four years in Philadelphia, which would probably have stretched out much longer if other institutions had not had their eye on him.

In Baltimore a new medical school was planned to accompany the newly opened Johns Hopkins Hospital. Johns Hopkins (1795–1873) was a bachelor who had made his fortune as an investor in the nation's first major railroad, the Baltimore and Ohio. His somewhat odd first name, "Johns," was his great-grandmother's maiden name.[7] Hopkins was a devout Quaker and fervent abolitionist who left $7 million of his estate to be divided equally to establish Johns Hopkins University and the Johns Hopkins Hospital. The former opened in 1876, followed by the latter in 1889 and the medical school four years later (it had been delayed in order to raise additional funds).

In 1889 John Shaw Billings recruited Osler from Philadelphia to Baltimore to become physician-in-chief of the new Johns Hopkins Hospital and professor of medicine at the medical school that opened in 1893. The Johns Hopkins School of Medicine represented a new era in American medical schools, with rigorous entry requirements and a strong emphasis on research, along the lines of the great German model that Osler and other leaders in American medicine admired. Candidates for admission to the new medical school were required to have a four-year college degree, including two years of premedical training in biology, chemistry, and physics, as well as a reading knowledge of French and German. Additionally, women were to be accepted as students—a relatively new twist in American medical schools at the time.[8]

From its inception the Johns Hopkins medical school had superb leadership. Once on board, Osler joined what has been called the Hopkins "Big Four"—the medical dream team of its day, with Osler in medicine, William S. Halstead in surgery, Howard A. Kelly in obstetrics/gynecology, and founding dean William Welch in pathology. Welch and his colleagues would build not only a new medical school, but the gold standard of medical schools in the United States. Joked Welch to Osler upon reviewing the tough student admissions criteria: "It was lucky we got in as professors; we never would have been able to go in as students."[9]

Osler picked up in Baltimore where he had left off in Philadelphia, as a clinician rapidly gaining international renown, who prided himself, above all else, in teaching students at bedside. From his Hopkins model of teaching evolved the clinical clerkship in which third- and fourth-year medical students work at the patient's bedside learning the art and the science of medical care. Osler considered bedside teaching essential for mastering the art of the physician, whose calling blended heart, mind, and hand. In late life he declared, "I desire no other epitaph . . . than the statement that I taught medical students in the wards, as I regard this as by far the most useful and important work I have been called upon to do."[10] For Osler, teaching in the wards was a distinction and the mark of a professional. The wards were the trenches. In them he demonstrated a love of the art and a mastery of the science that made the difference between treating a patient and treating a disease. Osler's specific advice to medical students attending the Albany Medical College in 1899 was, "Care more particularly for the individual patient than for the special features of the disease."[11]

Osler's brisk pace through the wards, accented with humor and non-stop teaching, guaranteed his popularity among students and faculty alike, while earning him stellar status as the physician's physician of the day. He invested himself in the full spectrum of the profession, from teaching, both at the bedside and in the lecture hall, to leading nationally through his personal involvement in professional organizations, some of which he launched himself and nurtured throughout his life. His humane approach to patients as individuals was a constant reminder to students and fellow physicians that medicine is a calling. In Osler's view, those who did not understand that medicine is an art as well as a science, and a calling, not a business, should seek other work.[12]

In his spare time at the hospital, Osler often ducked into a borrowed office, where he had amassed a mountain of books and notes. There he worked on a textbook that, when it was released by New York publisher D. Appleton and Company in March 1892, would be the medical textbook of its day. *Principles and Practice of Medicine* was reprinted through sixteen editions (the last in 1947) and eighty-four reprintings. Half a million copies sold during Osler's lifetime.[13]

The book made Osler an international name in medical circles and secured his financial independence for life. This enabled him to pursue his passion—building his personal library of 7,700 volumes into one of the world's great collections of medical books. Today it includes over eighty thousand books, manuscripts, archival materials, artifacts, and photographs housed at the Osler Library of the History of Medicine at McGill University in Montreal.[14]

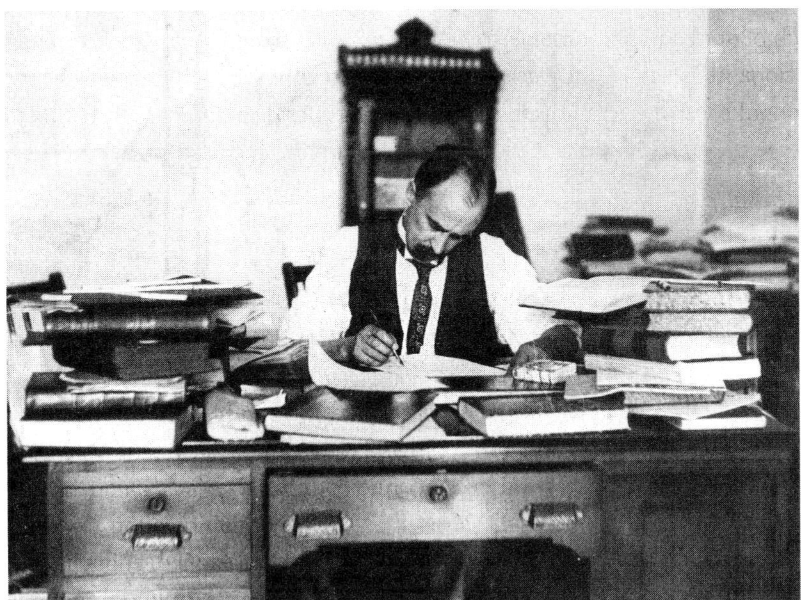

FIGURE 2.1. Sir William Osler writing *Principles and Practice of Medicine* at Johns Hopkins.

The first copy of the new textbook went to Grace Revere Gross (1854–1928), the widow of famed Philadelphia surgeon Samuel W. Gross (1837–1889). Osler had fallen in love with the widow, and while he was still toiling on his manuscript had asked her to marry him. A woman of strong will and purpose, she refused, advising him to finish the book before talking to her about marriage. Osler complied. He took the first signed copy of the soon-to-be-famous textbook to his bride-to-be, who was visiting friends in Baltimore, and delivered one of the most direct, no-nonsense proposals of all time—"There, take the darn thing; now what are you going to do with the man?"[15]

Grace Revere (the great-granddaughter of Paul Revere) accepted Osler's proposal at the doorstep and the two were wed four months later, in 1892. Their only son would be named Revere Osler (1895–1917).

Frederick Gates, a former Baptist minister and a trusted adviser to John D. Rockefeller (1839–1937), read Osler's new textbook from cover to cover while on a family vacation in the Catskill Mountains during the summer of 1897. Gates realized the book was something different. It brought into sharp focus how much new knowledge existed about the diagnosis of disease, yet how little was actually known about treatment. "To a layman like me demanding cures, [Osler] had no word of comfort," Gates would later write.[16] At Gates's urging, the Rockefeller Institute for Medical Research was created in 1901.

By 1905 Osler was a man worn thin by the stresses and demands of his work. Today we might label him as suffering from burnout. He had expended the vast energy necessary to familiarize himself with all the manifestations of his profession: he was physician, pathologist, historian, educator, author, bibliophile. And his scholarship was not limited to medicine. He was a Renaissance man with broad interests in history, literature, and world affairs, and he integrated these interests into his professional publications and even his innumerable commencement addresses. Moreover, as a leader in professional organizations, he was required to travel, speak, correspond, and generally hobnob. He bore the immense responsibility of being a principal spokesman for the medical profession. And his writing was so prolific that in his lifetime he produced 1,628 medical publications.[17]

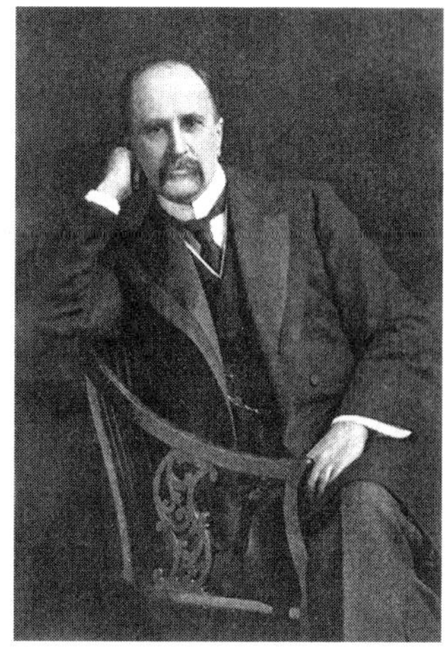

FIGURE 2.2. Sir William Osler in 1905.

And so, when on a visit to England in 1905 he was offered the Regius Professorship of Medicine by Oxford University, a distinguished position that would allow him to slow his pace, yet remain an international voice in medicine, there was no need to flip a coin. Osler's wife, like many of his medical colleagues, was concerned about the toll that his nonstop work habits were taking on his health. Upon hearing of Oxford's offer, Grace Osler immediately cabled her husband in England, "Do not procrastinate, accept at once. Better to go in a steamer than go in a pine box."[18]

As the Oxford Regius Professor, Osler had an international stage on which to solidify his reputation as the voice of the medical profession. Much in demand by universities and medical schools worldwide, he delivered commencement and keynote addresses that in and of themselves became well-worn books treasured by physicians to this day.

Osler's impressive home at Oxford, 13 Norham Gardens, is affectionately called "The Open Arms." There his latchkey approach to sharing his love of books and medicine persisted throughout his thirteen-year tenure, and students, faculty, and a constant stream of visitors, such as the poet Walt Whitman, would come. It was not uncommon for Osler to send Grace word in late afternoon that he would bring a few visitors by that evening for tea—only to arrive with fifty guests or more. Among them would be students, including a handful of Rhodes scholars like Wilburt Davison, who trained with Osler at Oxford and the clinics he organized at Radcliffe's infirmary. They would adopt Osler's humanistic approach to medicine and mentor future generations of physicians—including John P. McGovern—to take Osler's patient-centered approach to heart. And they would also take away with them memories of those wonderful evenings when Osler would pull a book from his library and delight in walking them through the pages of medical history. Here, day after day, they saw practiced the calling of medicine—a calling to which scholarship and love of life and people were central.

In 1911 William Osler, the boy who had been expelled from grade school in disgrace for his pranks, became Sir William Osler, a baronet, under King George V.[19]

Only six years later, Osler's worst fears about World War I and his only son's enlistment and service on the front lines in Belgium proved prophetic. Twenty-one-year-old Revere Osler suffered a fatal shrapnel wound from a German 4.2 inch shell.[20] Harvey Cushing, the neurosurgeon, happened to be nearby on the battlefront when Revere Osler was wounded. Cushing had been a resident at Johns Hopkins with his own latchkey to Osler's library, became a lifelong friend, and was to write a Pulitzer-Prize-winning biography about him. On hearing the news, Cushing hastened through the rain by ambulance to Revere's side at the 47 Casualty Clearing Station in Dozinghem. Revere, in shock and drifting in and out of consciousness, awoke to see Cushing and with a smile on his face said, "So glad you are here."[21]

Other eminent colleagues of the father came through the night and tried valiantly to save the young Osler, but to no avail. Revere Osler, the great-great-grandson of Paul Revere, died just before sunrise on August 28, 1917, and was buried in the Dozinghem Military Cemetery near Poperinge, Belgium, alongside more than three thousand other Commonwealth casualties of World War I.[22]

While Sir William Osler knew how to deal with death and grief after spending his lifetime in medicine, the loss of his only son was extremely difficult. On May 7, 1918, five months after Revere's death, Grace Osler wrote to Davison, her husband's former student at Oxford, about his grief:

> I am watching him very carefully. Since Revere's death he has grown very thin and his heart is simply broken—Oh—it is so hard to be cheerful and bear the disappointment and grief with a cheerful smile.
>
> I do hope this will not bother you but I know you won't mind trying to help the poor fellow.[23]

Despite this loss, Osler continue to work and look to the future—a testament to his character and to his resolve to make the most of every day. He would die on December 29, 1919, not of heartache over his son, but of bronchopneumonia and emphysema during the Spanish influenza epidemic. True to form, the man who personified the art of observation in patient care, the consummate teacher of medicine at the bedside, remarked to his friend and personal physician, Archie Malloch, "I've been watching this case for two months and I'm sorry I shall not see the post mortem."[24]

As a student of Osler and friend of the family, Wilburt Davison corresponded with Grace Osler throughout the nine years by which she survived her husband. In 1927, one year before Lady Osler's death at the age of seventy-four, Davison was selected as the founding dean of Duke University School of Medicine.

Back in Washington, DC, as the Great Depression brewed and Davison was building a new medical school, a young Jack McGovern was playing for all the marbles and putting his first seven dollars into his first savings account with aspirations of one day being a physician like his father. Little could Jack McGovern or Wilburt Davison know that they would soon cross paths.

Osler and Davison

Born in 1892 in Grand Rapids, Michigan, Wilburt Davison was the son of a Methodist minister. By 1913 he had received his AB degree from Princeton and was on his way to England to attend Oxford as a Rhodes scholar and to train with Sir William Osler. Over six feet tall and burly in build,

Davison was an imposing but jovial figure who adapted comfortably to his new college environment. He loved the Oxford rowing team and was socially as outgoing as he was scholastically adept.

But of course his studies, and particularly the opportunity to work with Osler, were foremost in his mind. "I first met Sir William Osler," he would recall later,

> during my first week as a medical student at Oxford. I had applied for permission to complete the first two years in one, but my Oxford tutor told me that "it isn't done," and sent me to 13 Norham Gardens, Sir William's home, hoping that he would immediately and definitely settle my nonsense.
>
> Instead, when Sir William met me at the door, he cheerily said, "I have been told of your request, which I think is very foolish, but of course you can do anything you please, and now let's have tea with Grace."[25]

Osler then went on to introduce Davison to Mrs. Osler with, "Grace, here is a new American colt who is wrecking a medical school tradition. Give him some tea."[26] Davison was so completely taken by the Oslers' charm that, he records,

> I soon felt that I had two friends at Oxford. My awe was immediately turned to adoration and affection.
>
> At the end of my first week at Oxford, and at other frequent intervals, he sent six or seven of us one of the following treasured invitations:
>
> *19 October 1913*
> From the Regius Professor of Medicine, Oxford
> *Dear Davison,*
> *If free, dine here with me Thursday evening, 23rd, 7:30.*
> *Sincerely yours,*
> *Wm. Osler*
>
> After dinner, he would bring out many of his precious books, which gave me a growing interest in medical history.
>
> Of Osler's many contributions to medicine, his greatest was his interest in students. His teaching was at the bedside and autopsy table. It was more

of an informal learning together than the didactic lectures at most medical schools before 1910.[27]

Davison thrived in the atmosphere Osler created. The great man took individual notice of students in the school environment as he did at his home, and treated them like colleagues in learning. Moreover, "Osler's interest in students commenced with their first year. He would dash into the anatomy, physiology and other laboratories, and address brief, amusing, or disconcerting questions or comments to each of us so that we felt, and correctly felt, that the 'Regius' was interested in us and in what we were doing."[28] Osler instructed in small matters as well as great ones, encouraging efficient time management and focus on the task at hand. It was Osler who quoted Thomas Carlyle to medical students, reminding them that "your business is not to see what lies dimly at a distance, but to do what lies clearly at hand."[29] Davison took these lessons to heart.

He would remember the privilege of driving Osler across the English countryside on weekly medical rounds. Other car trips resulted from Osler's reserve service as a lieutenant colonel in the Royal Canadian Medical Corps: "Every Monday during the first war, he would be driven to the Duchess of Connaught Canadian Hospital at Cliveden, Lady Astor's Estate. He usually took me with him to make notes for him. He would pile the week's medical journals on the seat between us. During these trips he would dog-ear the most interesting articles for me but I needed a week to read what he had covered in two hours."[30]

Davison took seriously his mentor's advice that research worth doing was research worth publishing. He followed this advice and later would see that medical students under his tutelage, students like John P. McGovern, did the same.

Osler suggested in 1915 that Davison should look into the growing number of cases of paratyphoid fever among British forces in the Dardanelles and Mesopotamia, especially those on hospital ships, where infections were passed from one patient to another. A paratyphoid vaccine was needed, and Osler and his Oxford colleagues felt that adding paratyphoid bacilli to the existing typhoid vaccine would have compounded benefits without interfering with the efficacy of the typhoid vaccine, as some insisted.

With Osler's direct support paving the way through complicated British paperwork, Davison acquired the license necessary for animal research. At the time, students in England were not allowed to lead such research, but Osler's students were special students, and Davison was allowed to proceed. The study was completed, and it verified the value of the mixed triple typhoid-paratyphoid A and B vaccine. The resulting work greatly reduced new cases of paratyphoid A or B fever, and Davison's thesis summarizing his findings earned him BA and BSc degrees, which were awarded by Oxford on May 11, 1916.[31]

With his Oxford medical studies completed, Osler recommended that Davison complete his medical degree at an American medical school and asked which one he would like to attend. A short note from Osler to Johns Hopkins medical school's dean William Welch was all it took to send Davison on his way to Baltimore and the Johns Hopkins University School of Medicine. There he completed his medical school requirements, trained in the renowned pediatric clinics of John Howland (1873–1926), and completed all the requirements for his medical degree. It was awarded the following year, in 1917.

Davison, who became a noted pediatrician, published his own textbook, *The Compleat Pediatrician*, in 1919, the year Osler died. Davison's textbook was originally developed as a notebook record of easily forgotten facts and methods. It weighed one pound for ease of carrying and stood a generation of pediatricians in good stead. Its practical, no-nonsense approach led to its being revised and reprinted many times over.[32] Davison learned to his great satisfaction that the book had been used after the surrender of Bataan to calculate the nutritional needs of American and Filipino prisoners of war.[33] John Bumgarner, a civilian physician captured by the Japanese early in the war, survived the infamous Bataan death march along with one of his few belongings—a well-worn copy of Davison's textbook. When Bumgarner found himself at Cabanatuan, a large POW camp north of Manila, the book was his only resource for diagnosing and attempting to manage the rampant nutrition-related diseases among his fellow POWs. His tattered copy is today on display at Duke.[34]

The textbook "would survive eight editions," as Davison was fond of saying, and he would offer a dime to anyone who found a typo or a fact in need of update. "I have a standing offer of a dime for every misspelled word and other mistakes . . . and the students and house staff find quite a number of them and make a small outside income." John McGovern, competitive and always up for a challenge, was the delighted recipient of more than a few of Dean Davison's silver Mercury dimes carefully taped inside letters over the years.[35]

Following his residency training, Davison returned to Johns Hopkins as a faculty member and assistant dean under Dean Lewis Weed. It was an administrative role he resisted at first but acquiesced to upon the advice of his pediatric chair, John Howland.

It is of note that pediatrics did not exist in Osler's time at Johns Hopkins. It became its own department seven years after Osler's 1905 departure to Oxford, with Howland appointed as founding chair. Howland emerged as one of the international stars in the young field and as a pioneer in the treatment and prevention of rickets and the discovery of a new fat-soluble vitamin his team would name Vitamin D. Needless to say, he was much sought after by Harvard and other medical schools, but he would remain a fixture at Johns Hopkins.

Howland's advice to Davison about adding the responsibilities of assistant dean to his pediatrics faculty role was simple and to the point. Davison recalled it years later: "[It] was to have two strings to my medical school bow given that some position might arise in which double training—administrative and pediatric—might be needed."[36] No doubt Davison understood that a position of leadership was essential if he was to open doors as Osler had opened them for him and so many others. A note from Osler had served as a medical-career hall pass anywhere in the world, and such authority came from a lifetime of leadership and respect. Davison added the assistant deanship at Hopkins to his patient-care duties under Howland.

The Duke University School of Medicine

The medical school at Duke was built on money derived from tobacco and hydroelectric power plants throughout the Piedmont region of the Carolinas. The two had made the family of James Buchanan Duke (1856–1925) a fortune many times over. The Duke family, known for their generosity, had a long history of using their wealth for the benefit of others, and improving the delivery of rural health care in the Carolinas (the area primarily served by their power plants) was very much on their minds.

The first attempt to establish a medical school in Durham had failed in 1892, the year Davison was born. In 1910 Dr. William Preston Few was elected president of Durham's Trinity College, and he soon renewed the attempt to establish the school. It took more than a decade and was fueled by many conversations with Governor Angus McLean and leading university and hospital presidents in the state. Even Abraham Flexner was involved in the discussion. It was Flexner who had published a famous report in 1910 challenging medical schools across the country to conform to models of excellence in teaching, patient care, and research, along the lines of Johns Hopkins.[37]

Few and James Buchanan Duke (1856–1925) connected in their thinking in 1924. Plans for Duke University were put on a fast track along with a commitment to launch a medical school. In December 1924, James B. Duke (Buck, as he was known) formalized the family's historic pattern of philanthropy by establishing the Duke endowment, a forty-million-dollar trust fund. The annual income was to be distributed in the Carolinas among hospitals, orphanages, the Methodist Church, three colleges, and a university built around Trinity College that would be renamed in honor of the Duke family.

Although Buck Duke died October 10, 1925, he left a codicil to his will dated ten days before his death and stating, "There is bequeathed to The Duke Endowment the sum of Ten Million Dollars and the Trustees shall use not exceeding Four Million Dollars in erecting and equipping at Duke University a Medical School, Hospital and Nurses Home."[38]

The Duke fortune is an interesting story in itself, one that dates back to 1865. On April 26 General Joseph Eggleston Johnston surrendered to Union forces led by General William Tecumseh Sherman at a farm near Durham known as the Bennett Place.[39] Durham was then a hamlet with fewer than one hundred inhabitants, and the post office was known as Durham's Station. The land had been donated by Dr. Bartlett Durham for building a railroad station, and the name had stuck. Partly because of the two-week delay in the Johnston-Sherman peace terms, due to General Robert E. Lee's surrender at Appomattox on April 9 and Lincoln's assassination five days later, the two armies remained camped in Durham with plenty of free time during the armistice. Free time permitted searching the countryside for the local tobacco found drying in barns.[40] The troops smoked all they could find. Upon their return, Union soldiers spread the word throughout the north about the exceptional quality of Durham tobacco.

Washington Duke, the patriarch of the Duke family, had been captured after the fall of Richmond. After returning to Durham he located a few barns containing tobacco that the Union soldiers had overlooked. Using a covered wagon, Duke and his sons James and Benjamin began filling orders that flooded in from the demobilized armies as they returned home.

The Duke family built one of the world's largest corporations (which included American Tobacco, Liggett & Meyers, R. J. Reynolds, and P. Lorillard). The town also was home of the first mill to produce denim and the world's largest hosiery maker. What had been a small town of five thousand in 1885 was by the 1920s a small city of forty-five thousand. It was during the early 1920s that James Duke and William Few embarked on a plan to add a medical school.[41]

Who would be better to get advice from about locating a dean able to build a medical school from the ground up, recruit faculty, and matriculate students, than the former dean of Flexner's model medical school, William Welch? Welch was the preeminent pathologist of his day and was considered by many in medical circles to be the dean of American physicians. He had built Johns Hopkins with Osler, served as the first president of the Board of Scientific Directors of the Rockefeller Institute for Research (he had been appointed in 1901), and remained a trusted advisor to Abraham Flexner. As president of the board at the Rockefeller Institute, Welch had recommended Abe Flexner's brother Simon, a former Johns Hopkins medical student, as the institute's first scientific director, a position Simon Flexner held for thirty-two years.

Davison remarked years later that when he originally read about the plans for a new medical school in Durham, he felt a bit jealous of whoever was going to get to lead it. At age twenty-six the young pediatrician and assistant dean at Johns Hopkins hardly thought he would be considered for the job:

> Needless to say I was amazed when Dr. Weed phoned me on 19 January, 1927, that Dr. Few was in his office and wanted to see me. The ensuing conversation with Dr. Few was characteristic of both of us—Dr. Few rarely going into details and I making rapid decisions. Few greeted me with, "I have come for you. Are you ready?" I replied, "Yes sir." Then he named the salary, the amount for building and for the endowment and asked whether they were satisfactory. I replied, "Yes sir." Few asked if I could start in September and I again replied, "Yes sir." He said he would ask the executive committee of the Duke University Trustees to confirm the appointment

> and that was the end of the interview. Two days later (January 21, 1927) I received a laconic telegram: "You have been elected. Delighted with prospect of working with you.—W. P. Few." My reply was: "Delighted with honor. Wish to express to you my great appreciation.—W. C. Davison."[42]

Sir William Osler would have been gratified to know that his young American colt was about to establish a medical school along the lines of Osler's beloved Johns Hopkins. Back in Oxford, Osler's widow, now seventy-three (and a year away from her death following a series of strokes), rejoiced at the news about Davison's new position. She expressed her satisfaction in the following note dated June 3, 1927, and addressed to "Jonah" (from Davison's Oxford days Grace Osler had called him by that name):

> I am greatly interested in this new scheme of life & future that you have taken on and send my most affectionate & sincere congratulations—for it means of course a reward for your hard work here and at the Hopkins—Dr. MacCallum was here and told me much of the plans for the new university. I hope you will not find the place too isolated—I would like to ask so many questions—but cannot on paper. Dr. Welch is in London and will come here next week and he will be able to tell one everything.[43]

Working around the clock, Davison set about building a medical school. He recruited the first faculty. As Osler had proclaimed, "Books are tools, doctors are craftsmen, and so truly as one can measure the development of any particular handicraft by the variety and complexity of its tools, so we have no better means of judging the intelligence of a profession than by its general collection of books."[44] With this in mind, on the day he was appointed Davison started building a library of medical books and journals. In his words, "They are more important than buildings, faculty, and students, and more difficult to find."[45]

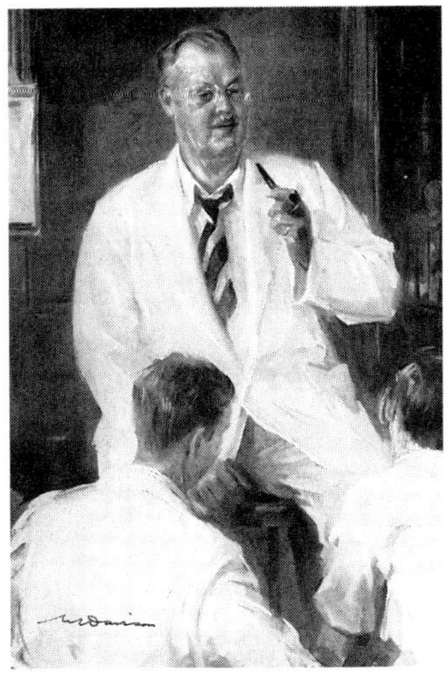

FIGURE 2.3. Wilburt C. Davison, McGovern's mentor and lifelong friend.

Mimeographed lists were compiled of the bound volumes of the Hopkins, Vanderbilt,

Rochester, and Boston medical libraries. They were sent to the fifty-seven leading book dealers around the world, from Tokyo to Stockholm, with a request for bids for delivery of any and all to Durham.[46]

Even on his summer vacations, Davison would scour bookstores in America and Europe and buy medical books at his own expense to give the library. "The biggest bargain was a complete collection of Leonardo da Vinci's drawings (28 volumes), similar to those which Osler had shown me in 1913, for $250 in Leipzig (Germany)."[47] In this way, Duke's medical library grew quickly to twenty thousand volumes at a cost of $227,000—a bargain by any measure, but especially given that many of these books are rare and now sell individually at auction for six figures or more.[48]

Simultaneously, ground was broken for the medical center in what was then a four-thousand-acre forest on the west campus, and faculty recruitment began. In the tradition of Welch and Osler's recruitment of faculty at Johns Hopkins, Davison sought chairmen who were relatively young and had tremendous promise. Osler, Welch, Kelly, and Halsted had started Hopkins at an average age of thirty-five. The average age for Duke chairmen appointed by Davison—thirty-five.[49]

Davison's recruitment methodology similarly followed the plan Johns Hopkins had implemented. Davison would select his first departmental chair in medicine (Harold L. Amoss) and the two of them would then pick the next chair, then the three would pick the next, until Duke had a full complement of outstanding faculty.[50]

On July 20, 1930, Duke University Medical Center opened to the public, followed by the medical school in October. It was a hot day, recalled Davison, who claimed he lost six pounds and ruined his new white linen suit showing visitors through the buildings. "The suit shrank so much that I gave it to a friend half my size."[51]

More than five thousand visitors from all corners of North Carolina attended the open house. Word of the new medical school attracted attention around the country, including in Washington, DC, where Mac McGovern and his young son took note through medical journals and newspaper headlines that something very special was happening to the south in Durham. It may come as no surprise that among the keynote speakers for the formal dedication of the new medical center, held on April 20, 1931, was none other than William Welch himself.[52]

The impressive and beautiful Duke campus, with its rolling, forested hills and its gothic buildings, provided the setting in which a new generation of medical students would study. They trained in an Osler/Davison academic environment where medical education included an appreciation of medical history and was facilitated by outstanding library resources and by clinical settings that integrated research with patient-centered care of the first order. It was an Osler/Davison setting made for McGovern.

Duke Undergraduate (1939–1942)

When Jack McGovern left Washington, DC, and headed 225 miles south to Duke, the medical school was a year away from celebrating its tenth anniversary. Already the school was turning heads in academic circles for the work of its innovative young dean and outstanding alumni. It was a school rapidly coming into its own as a fountainhead of bright new medical careers.

The arrival of a letter dated June 27, 1939, only six days after Jack's high school commencement ceremony, must have been an occasion for celebration in the McGovern household:

> *Dear Mr. McGovern:*
>
> *Your high school record and other recommendations qualify you for acceptance without entrance examinations into our freshman class. We wish for you a happy and successful college career and shall be happy to aid you in every way possible to achieve it. . . . If you should find within the time set for paying the fee that you will not be able to enroll here next September, please notify me immediately in order that the place now being reserved for you may be assigned to another.*
>
> *Sincerely,*
> *H. J. Herring,*
> *Dean of Men.*[53]

Needless to say, Jack, who had his eyes set on the premed program, wasted no time in reserving his spot—knowing full well that if he prospered in the undergraduate program, his chances of acceptance into the medical school would be good. Any earlier thoughts of attending Drexel University in Philadelphia were dropped by the wayside; Jack McGovern was Durham-bound.

One of Jack's friends as a freshman was Jay Maxwell, who years later recorded an early impression of him as "a wiry fellow whose natural voice often seemed about two decibels below a shout. He was always in constant movement and I guess his body was always in readiness for the next position it was to assume."[54] In an early letter to his father Jack provides a snapshot of his energetic and cheerful adjustment away from home for the first time: "Much water has gone over the dam since my last letter. At last we're under way! We have matriculated, bought our books, and received our gym assignments, our schedules, and tomorrow start classes."[55] That he had placed out of coursework in math and chemistry was a bit of good news to share with his parents back home, given his good, but not stellar, grades at Woodrow Wilson High, where he had fallen short of graduating in the top tier of his class.[56]

> They are putting me in the second year math class and best of all I'm skipping my first year chemistry and going right into "Qualitative Analysis." This means that I am able to take more math and more chemistry than most all the other pre-meds in four years. Only about 12 boys out of about 300 did this in chemistry. Father, old boy, I'm going to have to work my head off, as I not only have the tough medical course but am taking this advanced business. Don't worry though, I'll do it or bust! . . . Well, I'm going to develop a bit socially also. They will have dances, smokers [after all, this was Duke University, founded on tobacco money], and social gatherings of many sorts. I'm going to make it a point to attend some of these. . . . The food is good, I sleep fine, and I thank you again, as I always will for the splendid opportunity which you have spread before me.[57]

A month later—on October 21, 1939—in another letter home Jack reflected on the reality of the academic challenges ahead: "My roommate Tom is one of the naturally brilliant boys I have come into contact with. He plays around a great deal of the time, but gets excellent marks. He was first in his class in a high school of 3,000. I find that in comparison with other students, that I am above average intelligence, but not like Tom. I must work for what I get. I like to work though, so all is well."[58]

Throughout his life, McGovern would repeatedly demonstrate this drive and willingness to work hard, harder than others, if need be, to achieve success. He never perceived doubling up on effort as onerous; it was merely what you did to get ahead. College life proved highly congenial to him. From bonfires and football games to pledging with Pi Kappa Alpha (later he would add Phi Beta Kappa to his résumé), he loved the tradition and the camaraderie that a vibrant university like Duke could offer. He seemed to relish the recounting to his parents. On October 21, 1939, he writes:

> Dad, the last few days have been hectic. . . . this was home coming week. It's an old tradition at Duke to have a big bonfire (built of course by the freshmen), to celebrate the homecoming of the team. All the graduates attend this ceremony. All during the earlier part of the week, the freshmen work in afternoons building the largest bonfire you ever saw. It must be about 30 feet high. This isn't all there is to it however. As you no doubt know, the rivalry between Duke and North Carolina is keen, and they do everything in their power to get the laugh on us. Well, their aim in life about this time of year is to burn the Duke bonfire. In order to prevent this, the freshmen houses take shifts during the night to watch and guard the ever growing pile of wood. Everything went along fine Monday and Tuesday, and then on Wednesday our house had watch—I might add that I was on the shift from 1–4 in the morning. Nothing exciting happened Wednesday, but Thursday, with House P on guard, things began to pop. During the 1–4 watch, two boys came on with the regular P watch and said they were two engineering students from the East campus. The P boys fell for the ruse. The two boys were carrying a blanket and a black satchel which contained books, they said. . . . When the change in shift occurred at 4, the two boys went behind the fire, to the back of the woodpile, opened the black bag, and pulled out a can—I guess you can imagine what was in the can. Right, it was kerosene! The boys, who of course were from Carolina, lit the pile, and up in smoke went our labor. They made a clean get-a-way, the "rats."
>
> . . . So out we went to build a new one—on double quick. All went well, and last night, amid singing and cheering, Duke colors flew high before a mighty flame. At the fire, all the freshmen had to wear pajamas. It was the night of the pajama parade. After flitting about the fire like so many moths, we marched behind the band into Durham. On the way we would get on cars—as many as twenty on one car, no fooling! . . . Cheering and singing we marched thru Durham. We owned the town. At every intersection, we would sit down, stop traffic, and give a Duke cheer or song.[59]

And on March 22, 1940, he writes to his mother:

> Well, mother dear, Mrs. Burbank said that you will be unable to come down to get me [for Spring Break]. That is too bad, for I had refused several invitations to ride home. It probably isn't too late, and I may yet get a ride. If not I will come home via the "Seaboard Airline." I long to see you and dad again.
>
> Tomorrow is official "Hell day" for Pi K.A. pledges. We have to wear old shoes, our pants inside out, shirt on backwards, and in the evening we don't know what will happen. It is rumored that we are taken out in pairs and left about 50 miles from school, without money or any saleable articles. We must get back to school by morning somehow! Or else![60]

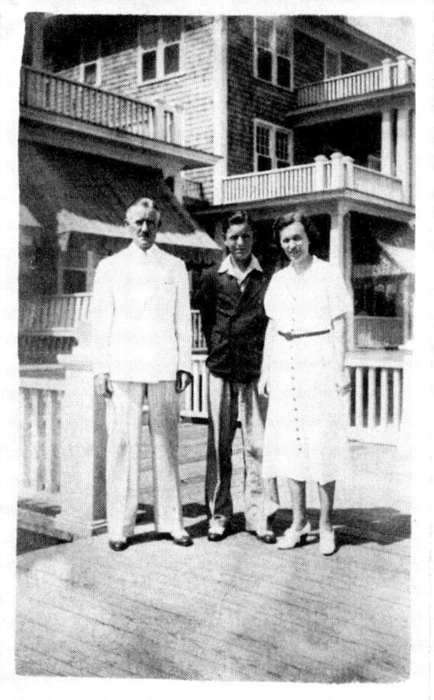

FIGURE 2.4. Jack as a Duke undergraduate vacationing with his parents at Ocean City, Maryland.

Back in Washington, the extended family of Browns, Hayeses, and McGoverns shared the letters and looked forward to the holidays, including spring break, when their college student would return home. Such good times contrasted with the ominous signs brewing in Europe of a second world war. During 1939 and 1940, his first year in college, Jack and the nation at large viewed the turmoil of Europe with apprehension—a collective dread that would flash into reality on December 7, 1941, just fifteen months into Jack's college education, with the tragic headlines of Pearl Harbor.

War concerns aside, college life at Duke continued on a high note, and the hard-working young McGovern progressed toward his goal of being accepted into a first-rate medical school—preferably Duke's, just over the hill on the University's west campus, where Wilburt Davison held sway. When McGovern had completed his two-year undergraduate premed studies, the time had arrived to formally meet Davison and make a case for being admitted into the medical program.

Medical School Days (1942–1945)

From the day Jack McGovern met Wilburt Davison, his life would change forever. The year was 1942, and Jack wanted passionately to get into Davison's medical school.

> I didn't know Dr. Davison in any way other than he was dean and this was the medical school I wanted to become a part of. During our first meeting, his confidence and casual attitude made me feel right at home and before I knew it I realized the Dean himself was interviewing me for a slot in the next class. In less than an hour I felt as if Dean Davison and I had known each other for years. He not only told me all about the Duke program he had established, he told me about his life and his mentor—a physician I had never heard of named Sir William Osler. I learned that Duke would train me to be a physician in the Osler tradition where medicine was a calling, not a business—I would be treating the whole person, not just the disease. I had a hundred questions to ask about this Osler tradition and Dean Davison, as busy as he was, gave me his time and his vision. I was hooked and wanted nothing more than to be accepted to Duke Medical School.[61]

At the end of the interview, Davison informed the anxious applicant that he was accepted into the incoming freshman class. The famous McGovern grin that his high school classmates had cited in his Woodrow Wilson yearbook no doubt stretched ear to ear when he heard those words of acceptance. At that moment, McGovern shook the hand that had shaken Osler's and was transformed in ways that mattered throughout his life. At that moment, McGovern's career began to gather around him.

Davison and McGovern would go on to be lifelong friends, as evidenced by the boxes and boxes of correspondence between the two for the next five decades.

When Jack's own father died young, Davison would become a surrogate father and a friend who could open doors with a phone call and serve as an experienced academic advisor—and a sounding board for Jack's racing mind, which could spew ideas like a geyser. In short, Davison's impact on McGovern, and thus Osler's, would be immeasurable.

Some sixty years after first meeting Davison, McGovern would remind students never to forget the people who had made a difference in their lives and had taken time to guide them and to open doors. Dean Wilburt Davison would always be at the top of McGovern's personal list, along with his wife, his parents, and his extended family of Hayeses and Browns.

Having spent the previous three years at Duke preparing himself for entry into medical school, Jack was well-liked and comfortable on the Durham campus and ready for the intensity of the accelerated pre-war medical training ahead of him. And he liked this dean of his and wanted to make an impression on him as a hard worker who would apply himself tirelessly to make the grade. Good was not good enough.

Making the grade at Duke in those early days when the medical school itself was barely a decade old meant finding your passion and pacing yourself. While Davison had built the school and curricula in the spirit of his Hopkins roots, he recognized that Durham was no Baltimore. While Duke had been referred to as the "Hopkins of the South," Davison never liked that identification and understood that the new environment of North Carolina required new methods of teaching.

The school had opened its doors on October 1, 1930, to the first class of seventy students. One of Davison's innovations was to establish a program at Duke that would allow students to proceed at a pace they set for themselves. In this way they could focus on the areas that attracted their interest and take only the fundamentals in fields they found less interesting. Therefore the faculty and the curricula were much more flexible than at many other medical schools. The trend of requiring a bachelor's degree for entry was also flexible. Davison felt that if a student fulfilled all requirements in his third undergraduate year, he should not spend a fourth year taking electives to fulfill the requirements for a diploma. Instead, those who entered the medical school without a bachelor's degree (as Jack did) could take a BS in medicine in addition to the medical degree if they distinguished themselves in research while completing the requirements of the latter.

This flexibility may seem less demanding on the surface. In reality, however, it proved effective in challenging students to set their own pace, identify their primary interests, integrate research into their work, and spend much more time in practical clinical rotations before graduating than many other medical schools of the day required.

At Davison's Duke, throughout the clinical years emphasis was given to patient follow-up, with teaching at the bedside. This Oslerian approach was considered more practical for teaching medicine than the alternative approach that called on students to spent more time in the lecture halls during their clinical years. As alumni would recall of their medical training during the 1930s and 1940s under Davison's program, its flexibility provided real opportunity to follow patients and review missed findings.[62]

The war years imposed upon Jack and his peers an accelerated three-year schedule for completing the medical degree. Success depended on enthusiasm for learning and ability to take advantage of the close working relationships among the faculty, house staff, and students. Students were forced not only to work hard, but also to learn and think on their feet. To add uncertainty to the students' situation was the fact that after Pearl Harbor and the United States' entry into World War II, military needs could invalidate student deferments.

One of Jack's classmates, Richard M. Paddison, recalled these unusual times:

> I remember Jack McGovern well as a friend and talented classmate in medical school, and that he was a good friend of Dean Davison's and always interested in pediatrics. When we were in medical school together it was wartime, and we were both in the Army Specialized Training Program (ASTP). This gave most of us more discretionary money than we had had previously, since the Army paid our tuition, bought our books, furnished our uniforms, and gave us $54 a month as Private First Class, as well as $3.50 a day commutation of quarters and rations. We were all forced to move out of the graduate dorms at that time, since there was an Army Finance School at Duke which crowded the undergraduate campus, and the undergraduates who remained were moved into the graduate dorms. Thus, those of us who were in the ASTP moved into apartments at various

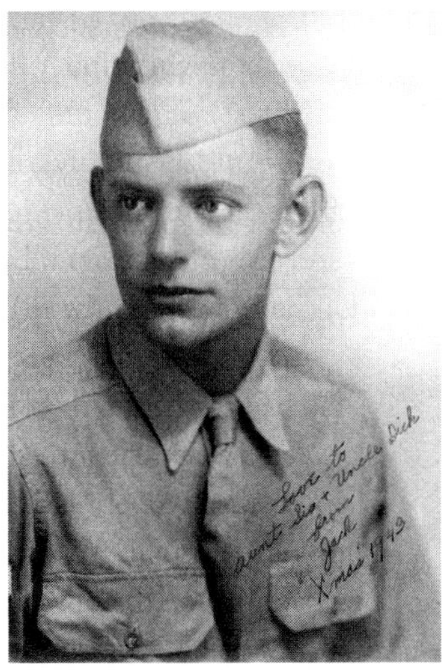

FIGURE 2.5. PFC McGovern, age 22, during his second year of medical school in the Army Specialized Training Program.

> locations in Durham. Communication between classmates was then a little more restrained than it might have been if we had all remained together in the graduate dormitories. The Class of '45 was the first accelerated class that graduated, and we were all assigned 9-month internships.[63]

Jack typically wrote his letters home late at night. He reflected on the day and reported on his progress. While the highest grades did not come effortlessly, his organizational skills and enthusiasm for work went into overdrive when they were needed and left few to doubt that this McGovern was a force to be reckoned with. Through it all, his love of medicine defined him, as his letters home demonstrate.

Letters Home—I Just Love This Medicine!

Throughout medical school, Jack's pace accelerated in response to the compressed curriculum and the uncertainties caused by the war. Exhausted as he might be from his self-driven quest to excel, his letters to his parents were alive with enthusiasm as he threw himself into the demands of medical school. To his father he wrote, in a letter dated "Sunday Morning 1944,"

> I am lost in the study of medicine for three years and there is no use denying it. I love it, and no one can convince me that there is anything more perfectly or more intricately organized than the human body. It is just like opening a novel with a good plot to it every time you take the covering off of the cadaver or take a squint through the "mike" [microscope]. I am really pleased. The work is hard, but I love it. The system down here is that you can set your own pace and no one watches over you. But you should see us fellows work.[64]

Student lockers were located in the school basement, and of the seventy-three members of McGovern's class, eight had last names starting with "Mc" and all of their lockers were together. On the first day of medical school, Jack met A. Ziegler McPherson, "Ziggy," as he was called by classmates. The two would become roommates, and the easygoing McPherson would prove a perfect foil for Jack's intense energy and drive. Ziggy had clear insights into his roommate's personality. "We began rooming together at the end of our freshman year when we were thinking about pediatrics as a specialty," he wrote later.

> Neither of us was of the "Jet Set," and we respected each other's freedom to study and live independently. Jack made friends readily and he was well acquainted with many of the medical students, as he had attended Duke University as an undergraduate. I was no match for him on the tennis courts. However, he found plenty of other students to play with in order to interrupt the labors of study. He must have studied Dr. Osler's teachings whenever he found the time.
>
> Jack's continuous drive in school was due to his own personality and character. . . . There are many persons who have their hobbies related to their professions. Jack is no exception. Medicine was his hobby in medical school, and it has continued to be his hobby as well as his profession.[65]

Looking back at their medical school days, Ziggy would remember another trait of young McGovern's that was in evidence many times over—a special business sense that later on could be tapped into for financial reward no matter how busy the man was as a physician. When the two roomed together off-campus for a year, they pitched in to buy a car jointly. Ziggy recalled that when they sold it they turned a small profit—thanks to Jack.

Jack's letters home from medical school have constant themes—they are about hard work and his love for his family, and about the world of medicine that was unfolding before him daily.

> *April 10, 1943—1:30 p.m.*
> *Dear Mother and Dad,*
>
> *This has truly been a tough week. I have truly never worked so hard in all my life, but believe we are really getting into the interesting things now. Wednesday night (11:30) I was called for my first autopsy. The body was of a 37 year old white female, para 1–0–1. She had had ademo-carcinoma of the uterus which had metastasized into most of her other organs. . . . The autopsy lasted til 3:30 a.m. The next twenty-four hours we had to have the autopsy report (clinical summary and protocol) written and passed in. Well, we went home and slept til eight o'clock and attended the 8:30 lecture. There were four of us in the group including "Ziggy." Then we had our regular Bacteriology lab to attend. In the afternoon we had our 1:30 lecture and afternoon pathology lab til five. We ate a hurried dinner and started on our protocol. We finished at 3:10 a.m. Thursday morning and passed it in. Got up at 8 and went*

through our normal schedule yesterday and last night worked til 12 a.m. in bacteriology. . . .

I am exhausted now and am going to jump in bed. . . . Learned more this last week than have ever learned in two weeks before. Boy, do I love this medicine!

Affectionately,
Jack.[66]

While other medical students were a bit apprehensive about their first autopsy, McGovern reported with delight the completion of his, including the challenge of working all night, getting to morning class, and finishing his report. The demanding nature of it all was for Jack thrilling—a test of mental and physical strength that he relished. Hard work in class, lab, clinic, and the wards was a constant.

Vacations were few and brief, clouded by the turmoil of World War II and the change it brought to familiar peacetime routines. To break the cycle of work and study, tennis now replaced Jack's childhood love of sandlot baseball. It was a competitive sport that would prove to be a great stress reliever; he used it for years to come. Always interested in others and popular on campus for his enthusiasm and his grin, he could often be found in his leisure hours at a local beer and barbecue stop known as Turnages—which, with its low ceilings, well-worn tables and beer mugs, Carolina charm, and tasty barbeque was universally popular among the students. Jack frequented it whenever extra time and change in the pocket would allow.[67]

On April 13, 1944, he wrote home about a new experience:

I had my first delivery Wednesday at 7:05 p.m. She was a para 3–0-3, 29, m, w, f. I stayed up with her 36 straight hours watching the progress of her labor, taking fetal heart rates, observing the gradual effacement of the cervix, taking B.P.'s, giving fluids per I.V., etc. She had a breech delivery and had a tough time of it. The nurses brought me food. The patient said that if she had a little boy that she was going to name it John Phillip or J. P., nicknamed Jack. I told her that this was no way to give a boy a good start in life (kidding her). Well, needless to say it was a little girl.[68]

While Jack did not get his first delivery named in his honor, he did pick up some key insights during it that reinforced his desire to train in pediatrics.

> Watching my first delivery (at the beginning of the quarter) gave me a great thrill. The first thought that went thru my mind was how in hell mothers could give birth without the aid of a physician. It looked like a full-sized job for any man to me, but it just once again proves how nature can get along pretty well a great deal of the time without us physicians. We get to think we are so red hot, at least many of us, but old mother nature will do a great deal if left alone. I am already developing a conservative attitude towards "Rx" except where unquestionably indicated. Of course, the big job is to learn enough so as to know what to do and be right—theory is a must for the background for that knowledge, but the combination of that theory with a good practical cerebration can't be beat.[69]

In this way, through his own observation and training Jack was coming to accept an article of wisdom that his father had always preached while recounting tales of Walter Reed and Garfield hospitals during the depression years: a little "horse sense" goes a long way for any physician.[70] He was also about to learn a lesson from Dean Davison's preachments on the value of doing research.

Winning the Borden

In the tradition of Osler, Dean Davison insisted that integrating research into clinical work was essential. To make research more interesting, the student who conducted and presented the best research during the final year of medical school would be recognized at graduation as winner of the Borden Prize, with a cash award of $500. It was a coveted prize that would distinguish one student from all others, and if the research was exceptional, it might lead to a bachelor of science degree in addition to the medical degree. Jack took to the challenge with a zeal and tireless passion that surprised even those of his peers who outperformed him in the classroom with much less investment in their studies.

The Borden prize in medical research was offered to medical schools throughout the country. Its purpose was to challenge the best students to identify and carry through with an original research project considered by each school as the best student project of the senior year. The $500 in prize money was not nearly so valuable to most students as the recognition and personal satisfaction of winning the Borden.

The founder of the Borden Prize was an interesting fellow. Gail Borden Jr. (1801–1874), born in Norwich, New York, had been a surveyor and schoolteacher in Mississippi before going to Galveston, Texas, in 1829. There he further diversified his skills as a farmer, a surveyor for Stephen F. Austin's colony near San Felipe, and a newspaper publisher (of the *Telegraph and Texas Register*).[71] He then added to his credentials by becoming a real estate agent, helping sell lots on Galveston Island. By 1837 Borden was in Houston surveying the original lots of the new city that had been built along Buffalo Bayou two years after the first topographic map of Texas had been compiled.[72] He also served as the first tax collector of the Port of Galveston under the Republic of Texas, a position he resigned following a dispute with President Sam Houston.[73]

A century before Jack McGovern entered Duke Medical School, Galveston had suffered through a serious epidemic of yellow fever. An entrepreneur at heart, Borden experimented unsuccessfully with large-scale refrigeration as a means of preventing the disease. His attempt to develop a meat biscuit made of dehydrated meat compounded with flour[74] also failed, but his next idea took the nation by storm.

In 1853 he sought a patent on a process for condensing milk in a vacuum. Meat biscuits were out, but condensed milk was a hit and proved a huge success in the late 1850s, a time when the Civil War created great demand for such a portable and long-lived product. Factories in Connecticut and New York brought Borden great wealth, and from that wealth and his interest in challenging future inventors through research emerged the Borden Prize. That Gail Borden had left New York for Texas because of a persistent cough that no doctor of the day could tame made medical research all the more important to him. For Jack, winning the Borden Prize in research was high priority, and little could stand in his way once he seized upon his subject. Gail Borden would no doubt have been pleased that young McGovern selected a cough for his research—whooping cough.

Whooping cough, *pertussis,* is caused by the bacterium *Bordetella pertussis* and is highly contagious, spread by contact with droplets expelled in coughing or by contact with hard surfaces contaminated by the droplets. The bacteria localize and thrive in the lining of the lungs, where they produce toxins that damage the tiny hairs or cilia of the lungs. This results in an increased inflammation of the respiratory passages and the typical dry cough that produces a deep "whooping" sound as the patient tries to take a breath. Whooping cough is contagious from seven days after exposure to the bacteria and up to three weeks after the onset of coughing spasms. The most contagious time is during the first stage of the illness.[75]

It was in 1906 that Jules Bordet and Octave Gengou first isolated *Bordetella pertussis* bacteria in pure culture.[76] By the 1920s, a vaccine for whooping cough was developed. In the 1940s, as Jack McGovern entered medical school, more than five thousand deaths from whooping cough were reported annually in children under the age of six months in the United States, yet immunization against the disease was not administered until six months.[77] Jack realized that a study of immunizations conducted on infants of two or three months was needed.

The results would be measured by using post-immunization sera with an innovative mouse protection test technique. For this Jack would need research space, mice, and Dean Davison's approval. Typical of Jack's often hyperactive enthusiasm, he notified the dean that he had an "emergency situation to discuss" and needed an appointment "just as soon as possible."[78]

In this way Jack's senior Borden project was launched. His intensity and his all-out attack on the research questions at hand left an indelible impression on his classmates, who remember the tireless, around-the-clock effort he invested. Hilda Pope Willett, a Duke graduate student in the Microbiology Department at the time and Jack's research assistant, wrote later about his approach to the project.

> Dr. David T. Smith, Chairman of the Microbiology Department, provided the laboratory space and basic microbiologic supplies. It was Dr. Smith who recommended me to Jack to care for his experimental mice. As a brand new graduate student in the Microbiology Department, the five dollars weekly remuneration that Jack offered me was a welcome addition to my $75 monthly stipend, and compensated for the menial nature of the task. I gladly accepted the offer.
>
> Jack believed in the work ethic; his conscientious attention to his senior medical rotations usurped all of his daytime hours. It was only in the late evening that he found the time for his research, beginning when most others were quitting for the night. With dogged persistency of purpose, however, night after night he would return to the lab for work on the pertussis project. As time went on, he began to draw more and more on my assistance, and very rapidly the job of "mouse-keeper" expanded in scope, and

> Jack accepted me as a colleague and co-worker. We spent many enjoyable hours working together on the pertussis experiments, discussing results, and planning the next experiments. During this period he appeared indefatigable, working long exhausting hours as if driven by some superhuman force. Never was there one word of complaint or self-pity. He set his own goals and priorities and worked diligently to attain them. Never did he leave me to finish an experiment alone because he was too fatigued to continue, although many times he did appear on the verge of complete exhaustion.
>
> It is not the scientific brilliance of that research project that I remember most today, but the enthusiasm and eagerness with which he approached it. Jack's enthusiasm was contagious, and soon I too was caught up in it. . . . The Dean served to kindle and keep ablaze in Jack the tremendous enthusiasm he exhibited in every facet of his life. After a single meeting with the Dean, no obstacle was insurmountable. It was through these conversations that there also emerged a picture of Jack as a person, his humaneness and basic character. Jack was one of the most forthright persons I have ever known. His frankness was disarming and immediately created a feeling of mutual trust and confidence. Unlike many individuals with high personal aspirations and goals, Jack always had time for other people and was exquisitely considerate of the feelings of others.[79]

Hearing of his son's research project to win the Borden Prize, Mac McGovern offered his own fatherly encouragement as a surgeon who admired good research but had never invested himself in research per se. On August 19, 1944, Mac wrote to his son, "Glad to hear your report that your experiment is progressing to your satisfaction and hope that it ultimately will accomplish what you hope for. . . . Whether it turns out fruitfully or not, it has been a worthwhile undertaking for you, is directly in line with your clinical medical training and gives you a firsthand practical understanding of adventures in medical research. . . . So, son, stay with it to the extent that it is compatible with your regular curriculum."[80]

Jack won the 1945 Borden Research Prize with his paper, "Passive Intraperitoneal Mouse Protection Test in a Study of Immune Response to H. pertussis Vaccination." A copy of the $500 check, a handpicked memento of what was among his proudest lifetime accomplishments, can be found in his personal scrapbook. Next to it is a handwritten note from Dean Davison: "The Borden Company has just presented the Medical School with a beautiful bronze plaque with the names of the winners of the Borden Award. I am very happy that your name leads the list."

It is interesting to note that in more recent times whooping cough, like so many infectious diseases, was considered nearly conquered and a problem of the past. But on April 3, 2012, the disease was declared an epidemic in Washington State by the Centers for Disease Control and Prevention—a development McGovern would no doubt find of great interest.[81]

The experience was a game changer for the budding new physician, who would forever integrate original research into his work.

The resolute preoccupation with work at hand that Hilda Willett saw in Jack during the Borden project would follow him throughout his career and could be detrimental to people closest to him, despite Willet's assertion that he "always had time for other people and was exquisitely considerate of the feelings of others." One egregious example occurred when Jack's parents drove the two hundred miles from Washington to Durham early that busy senior year to take him Thanksgiving dinner. What had always been a highly anticipated annual event for the family turned out to be a major disappointment to father and mother, who now found themselves competing with their son's research for his attention. They ended up sharing most of the Thanksgiving dinner at Jack's off-campus apartment with his roommate, Ziggy. Winning the Borden left little time even for those who cherished Jack's presence the most.

Despite an apologetic letter from Jack some days later, Mac McGovern could not resist expressing his disappointment at having had to dine with a roommate while Jack tended to his mice and his research.

December 8, 1944
Dear Jack:

I have no doubt that you have been anticipating this letter from us. It is overdue but the days skip by. . . . I must admit your mother was a bit more worried than disappointed. She remarked to me, and she was 100% right that she thought that you did not react as might have been expected of you, on the occasion and all circumstances well considered. I am glad that you admitted this fact in your letter and that you offered an explanation therefore. I had pondered in my own mind for a rational explanation. I suggested to Lottie that your routine work plus the unusual effort you were putting into your research had made you a bit preoccupied. Surely she was disappointed as she had done a real job; she forgot nothing; her thoughts were entirely of you and making Thanksgiving happy and pleasant for you. . . . Leaving DC at the time was not at all convenient for me. Oct, Nov. and December are my busiest times but I could not resist your mother's altruistic desire and genuine eagerness to see you, your apartment, Thanksgiving Day Dinner with you. . . . both your mother and your dad were righteously a bit disappointed and let it go at that[,] for your explanation, while it is plausible is to say the least, not very weighty.

To both your mother and I you are an inspiration; a son we point to with humble pride and satisfaction, ever living to see you do greater and greater things, which I know will find you a place in the profession of your choice that we will be proud of and in which you will surely find a fruitful life of contentment, satisfaction, and happiness. Hope you are well, write when you can.
Affectionately yours,
Dad.[82]

Mac had observed the ability of his son to put everything, even parents, aside for the sake of personal ambitions. It was a trait Jack would do his best to harness throughout his life, but his driven passion for work at hand would almost always break loose.[83]

Despite this lamentable incident, Jack was in fact deeply grateful to his parents and he expressed his gratitude openly and throughout their lives. His letters to them show an understanding of their investment in him of time, love, and imagination. The letters also show an awareness of his parents as people with their own identities; he demonstrates a touching sensitivity to their small vanities. On the occasion of their twenty-fifth wedding anniversary he wrote them a letter expressing his certainty "that no son was ever exposed to a finer more wholesome or honest environment," and then breaks off from praising Mac and Lottie as parents, for a reason somewhat surprising, perhaps, in a twenty-two-year-old: "I could go on and enumerate all that you have done for me, but this is not the place for that. This is your day, Mother and Dad."[84] He is acknowledging that his parents have a life outside of their life as his parents.

Transitions

Both father and mother, along with Aunt Sis and her husband, Ed Nevils (Uncle Dick to the family), were front and center at Jack's graduation from Duke University School of Medicine in Page Auditorium on the morning of Saturday, June 23, 1945. Mac sent his son the plan. "Talked with Uncle Dick last Tuesday. He and Aunt Sis want to attend your graduation. They would go in my car . . . hence I am anxious that you try and arrange for a minimum of baggage so that we can all come home together. Can't you box and express a great deal of your effects?"[85]

Graduation was for Mac a moment of great paternal pride. On May 20, 1945, he wrote his son a letter of congratulation:

> The final hurdle, your private examination by the three faculty members was indeed a triumphant and fitting climax for the overall effort that you had put into your undergraduate and graduate education. To take on the extracurricular work that you did in an already stepped up program was more than courageous. That the University saw fit to acknowledge your accomplishments by awarding you the B.S. . . . [is] an attainment of which you can well be proud, and for which, I sincerely assure you, your mother and I are more than proud. As you are well aware, I have never been one to "yes" everybody; to become unduly elated at my own efforts and to go out of the way to pile praises upon one for normal work done. But, here you took on a great deal more than was normally expected of you; you stuck to it; saw it through and although discretionary on their part the faculty saw fit to appraise your effort, stamped it with approval and duly rewarded you. How could any father but feel elated over such accomplishments of his son.[86]

On graduation day, Jack McGovern joined his seventy-three Duke classmates (only two of whom were women, as was common at the time) reciting the Hippocratic oath, led by Dean Davison, and became John P. McGovern, MD. He graduated with his medical degree, a bachelor of science in medicine (one of three in his class to accomplish this added feat), and special recognition as the school's first recipient of the Borden Undergraduate Research Award in Medicine. He also graduated with a commission as a US Army first lieutenant in the Corps Reserve. All but two in his graduating class held commissions in either the Army, the Navy, or the US Public Health Service—a sign of the times during these war years.

On the advice of Dean Davison, he would leave his beloved Duke to do a year of residency training in pediatrics at Yale in New Haven, Connecticut. The dean wisely suggested that the change in scenery to a new medical setting would broaden and enrich the postdoctoral training experience. McGovern had an agreement with him to return to Duke after one year to complete his residency. A complicating factor was the uncertainty of the ongoing war; all of the commissioned graduates in McGovern's class faced the possibility of being called to active duty.

McGovern had already made clear to his father that he was prepared for whatever was required. In a letter dated May 25, 1944, he writes:

> My views on "Americanism" completely coincide with yours and at any time that I would be called on to do my all to protect our freedom I would do so willingly. I also feel my obligation to do my share as an enlightened citizen to see that we have good, clean, honest government. We Washingtonians are rather limited, however, not having a vote, but at best as a physician I shall join and support the AMA and my local society and do my best to see that our profession is saved from regimentation by self-serving politicians.[87]

Jack McGovern had reached the pinnacle of his childhood dream and was now a newly minted Duke physician. Throughout his life, his parents had provided every opportunity and unconditional support to help him achieve his aspirations. His father had served as a role model for the profession and for leading day-to-day life. Many of the letters from father to son are peppered with reminders to pay attention to such details as eating well, resting, watching over the mechanical condition of the car—there was even a reminder to check the antifreeze and park in a safe spot when away from Durham during the holidays.[88]

In many ways, father and son had much in common, but they were on divergent life paths, the one leaving medicine and the other entering the profession. Mac had good reason to be concerned that his son take care of his health. As Jack entered his final year of medical school, Mac learned he had tuberculosis.

Only a year earlier, in 1944, Mac had been named chief of surgery at Garfield Memorial Hospital and elected president of the medical staff. Now his diagnosis darkened his proudest moment as his son completed his medical degree. The year that Jack graduated from medical school, Mac announced his retirement to shocked colleagues. Colonel A. C. Gray spoke for the District of Columbia Selective Service System when on Oct. 2, 1945, he wrote to Mac, "Your letter of resignation, as a member of Appeal Board Panel No. 4, addressed to Mr. Leahy came as a great surprise and a real shock to me. I am truly sorry to learn of your illness and sincerely trust that it will not be long before you are entirely restored to health."[89] This was one of nearly thirty letters representative of the community-wide sense of surprise and sadness upon news of Mac's ill health.

For Jack, the announcement was the culmination of nagging concerns he had harbored about his father's health throughout his years at Duke. Writing to his father shortly after beginning medical school with the bold proclamation, "I just love this medicine!," he almost buried his real cause for writing, using the very last inch of the last page to add, "P.S. Have quit smoking again father, Have you quit drinking?"[90] Many years later, in a 1998 oral history interview at Baylor College of Medicine, he would reflect further on struggles with alcohol and tobacco, saying, "I had seen so much of a problem in practice of alcoholism and drug abuse. I had seen so much of the problem with my colleagues in medicine, and I think I saw it in my own home. They didn't call it alcoholism then. My dad was a periodic drinker. It would be just one night and he'd change totally. But all of his brothers did. They all drank and smoked Camel cigarettes, and died pretty young. The two sisters didn't drink at all and lived to old age."[91]

Following his tuberculosis diagnosis, Mac would be diagnosed with hepatitis and suffer a prolonged decline in health that would cast a pall over the first six years of his son's postgraduate education (1945–1951). Mac's failing health required that Jack assume a constant watch over his parents' well-being while completing some of the most rigorous years of his own professional development. The choice of Yale and New Haven for his residency provided more than an important training opportunity away from Davison and Duke—it also put the young physician in the Northeast, with more convenient transportation to Washington, where his aging parents still lived.

But within a few short years the family home at 3601 Cumberland would be rented, and his parents would move into a cottage in Braddock Heights, a country suburb of Washington, located in Frederick County, Maryland. Here they would find a house in a much quieter and more restful neighborhood that, Mac would report to his son in Durham, was most acceptable: "This little cottage that we have could not be better. It is beautifully located and has all the comforts necessary and what is more important, I am perfectly happy up here. Resting, i.e. relaxing better than I ever. . . . My back screened in porch overlooks the Valley which you will remember is really healthful"[92] (May 1946).

During the new Dr. McGovern's postgraduate trainings years, letters from father to son no longer recounted details of a busy surgeon's patient outcomes or of political battles fought for the DC Medical Society and the profession. Now the letters were chronicles of the father's sufferings from mounting health problems, the outcomes of continual medical tests, impending medical appointments and procedures, and continual dental problems requiring what Mac referred to as calls upon "the tooth carpenter."[93]

The surgeon/father had become now the father/patient, and Jack would now and forever after view medicine through the patient's eyes. Osler's timeless advice to care for the patient, not the disease, could not have hit home more directly. The father who had once written his son letters filled with professional advice now wrote letters that invoked concern and worry: "Mother and I went to DC last Wednesday, Thursday. I had five (5) lower teeth extracted, X-rayed (chest), fluoroscope, blood count and sed rate. Peabody was pleased with my progress. The teeth had been bothering me considerably"[94] (August 19, 1946).

But despite Mac and Lottie's difficulties, they did not turn all their attention inward; they continued to be interested in their son's life, inquired into it, commented on it, expended imagination on it.

Mac McGovern died on July 28, 1951, at Mount Alto Hospital in Washington, DC.[95] Supported by a steady stream of letters of condolence, including touching tributes from Mac's colleagues and Dean Davison at Duke,[96] mother and son oversaw Mac's burial with full military honors at Arlington National Cemetery. Seventeen years later—in 1968—Jack would still feel the loss of his father and would reflect on it in a letter to Lottie:

> As I write this today I know that it is October 30 and would have been yours and Dad's golden wedding anniversary. How much I miss him and how often I think of him, which is daily, as his picture is in front of me on my desk and on my wall. He is forever in my mind and heart, just as you are, dear Mother. I hope that it didn't rain so that you were able to take over the chrysanthemums to his grave in Arlington National Cemetery as you had planned. I recall that he always sent you chrysanthemums on your wedding anniversary.[97]

The loss of his father, though long dreaded and clearly foreseen, was difficult for McGovern, who for the rest of his life would honor the memory of the man who had led him by the hand through the corridors and crowded wards of Garfield Hospital and who had died so lamentably young. But the close friendship and mentorship of Davison helped to soften the blow. And McGovern would find renewed support and guidance from his former dean for another twenty years.

Lessons in Mentorship—The Second Father

Dean Wilburt Davison, Osler's American colt, would become the father figure, friend, confidant, and mentor that Jack's father could no longer be for him as he went through his key postgraduate and professional development years. Davison saw in his friend and former student a man young, hard-driving, and committed, who was clearly going places. Jack's life and many accomplishments after the death of his father were profoundly influenced and shaped by Davison and constitute a textbook example of the two-way street that defines true friendship and mentorship.

Mentoring is an essential process in transferring key elements of professionalism in medicine. Davison as role model was no less essential than lectures and textbooks to Jack McGovern's development as a physician, scientist, and humanitarian.

The origin of the word "mentor" lies in mythology. Mentor was the friend in whose hands Odysseus, king of Ithaca, left his infant son Telemachus and his wife Penelope when he sailed away to wage war on the Trojans. It was Mentor who was responsible for Telemachus's education as well as for the shaping of his character, the wisdom of his decisions, and the clarity and steadfastness of his purpose. Mentor was the key figure in Telemachus's life on his journey from youth to manhood.[98]

Davison was McGovern's Mentor. Davison's intellectual style, professional priorities, deliberateness, truthfulness, and even his approach to personal relationships were translated into the daily style and outlook of the young McGovern and many other Duke-trained physicians. Davison also transferred academic character through the daily habits he modeled in the program he had established at Duke. Inspired by Davison's example, McGovern went on to further develop and fine-tune his own ideas about scholarliness, lifelong learning, thoroughness, and respect for the art and science of the medical transaction.

And Davison was of course himself to a large extent the product of Osler's mentoring. Summarizing what Osler represented, Davison identified Osler's strengths through seven distinct roles: as a physician, teacher, scientist, medical reformer, medical writer, humanist, and personality with lasting presence. In Davison's words, "We must demonstrate to this generation not only what he was and meant to us, but what he did for them and for medicine, and can continue to do if the medical youth will try to emulate him as we attempted to do. He embodied, applied, and transmitted all that is the finest and best in a physician."[99]

Osler and Davison made McGovern possible. Together they forged a professional path that McGovern followed at high speed and with a success that dazzled even Davison.

Chapter Three

Pediatrician and Allergist

DURING OSLER'S DAY more than a century ago, physicians were typically generalists; today's many specialties had not yet come into being. Osler was known as "The Chief" at Johns Hopkins, and his responsibilities encompassed all medicine.[1] William Halsted led surgery, Dean Welch commanded pathology, and Howard Kelly oversaw obstetrics. That was it. Four chairmen with their supporting faculty covered all the needs of teaching medicine to some of the best and brightest medical students the nation had to offer. But by the 1940s, when McGovern was training at Duke, specialization was rapidly on the rise and specialty boards were being created to develop and enforce practice standards for them.

The concept of a specialty board to set standards for the ongoing evaluation and certification of physicians was first proposed in 1908 by Derrick Vail (1864–1930) in his presidential address to the American Academy of Ophthalmology and Otolaryngology. While there is some dispute whether Vail or his colleague Edward Jackson deserves the credit,[2] ophthalmology did in 1917 become the first specialty to form a board. By 1933 the first three specialty boards (for ophthalmology and otolaryngology, dermatology, and obstetrics and gynecology) formed the Advisory Board of Medical Specialties, today known as the American Board of Medical Specialties (ABMS).[3] That same year pediatrics joined the growing list of specialties.

By comparison, in 2012 the ABMS oversaw twenty-four medical specialties, encompassing more than one hundred subspecialties. Clearly medical students now face growing complexity in choosing and preparing for certification in a field.[4]

McGovern's medical training at Duke was directly affected by the events at Pearl Harbor and the formal entry of the United States into World War II on December 8, 1941—he and his classmates at Duke found themselves on the special three-year accelerated undergraduate program discussed in the previous chapter. This left them less time to determine their specialty interests. But while many of his classmates struggled over choosing a specialty, McGovern studied the options and found pediatrics a natural fit. He reminded his father that even as a boy following him around Garfield, he had always gravitated to the newborn window to look at the babies, and added, "Well, believe it or not at my age I still like to go look at them. I sneak into the nursery at night and look them over quite often. Watching my first delivery gave me a great thrill"[5] (April 13, 1944).

Abetting McGovern's decision to pursue pediatrics was the fact that Dean Davison was a pediatrician and author of one of the key textbooks in the field at that time. Also, of course, McGovern had chosen his undergraduate research project to address whooping cough in infants, and having won the Borden Prize was a credential in pediatrics not to be dismissed.

While pediatrics and the growing field of allergy and immunology would be McGovern's choice for his lifework in medicine, like all students he did explore other specialties during his clinical training. Writing to his father during his senior year, he minced no words about his initial impression of psychiatry, although it was one that would change significantly over time:

> You asked what my reaction to Psychiatry was and so I'll give you that first. I have been on Meyer Ward ("the nut factory") now for 5 days and have already read a small psychiatry book thru from cover to cover. My interest in psychiatry is, however, only in the theoretical connotations involved and I play at it more as a game than anything else. . . . I consider 60% of it plain and simple "bull shit." I firmly believe that there is really a place for the sound psychiatrist and interested research worker, but they have a long way to go yet. Let me know what you think in your next letter. I wouldn't be a psychiatrist for $1,000,000 however.[6]

McGovern's fond memories of his childhood pediatrician R. V. Mattingly also apparently influenced his interest in medicine and perhaps in pediatrics, despite his father's own specialty of surgery. Upon learning from his mother of Dr. Mattingly's death in 1970, he wrote her that he "was greatly saddened" by it. "He, Dr. Jansen, Dr. Ong, and Dr. Walker got me through the childhood diseases and, of course, I vividly remember each of them. No doubt each, along with Dad, played a part in my decision to go into medicine."[7]

By the age of fourteen McGovern was already patterning his outlook on a career in medicine from the role models he knew best. He cited both his father and R. V. Mattingly in the bibliography of the junior high school paper in which he proclaimed his interest in medicine as a vocation.[8] Their examples had acquainted him with the time, money, and effort necessary to qualify for a career in medicine, and also with the inconveniences attendant on the profession:

> The doctor renders a vital service to his community, and must be on the job, in rain or shine—night or day, to perform his mission of healing. His life will be irregular—his eating, his sleeping. In all possibility his income will be low. But the personal satisfaction he will receive, if he is a man of the right caliber, will duly compensate for his sacrifice.
>
> . . . There are years of toil and sacrifice ahead of the young man, who starts out to become a physician, and only inspiring and abiding devotion to his work can keep him persistently at his task until he reaches his goal . . . If he intends to specialize (much specialization has come into medicine in the past 50 years), one or two more years of graduate work will be necessary, requiring with it more money and time.[9]

It seemed to McGovern that accomplishing something truly beneficial for the welfare of humanity was central to a good life. Treating children qualified. It gave him a satisfaction from which he never allowed his medical career to stray far. It was clear to those who observed him on student rounds that pediatrics was his primary interest. As a medical student under the influence of the pediatrician Davison, he plunged into the pediatrics wards at every opportunity and reported to his parents about the experience: "I have spent a great deal of the last week on Pediatrics (from the standpoint of physical diagnosis). This has been a most enjoyable experience for me as I really love the little brats and they seem to have a great deal of confidence in me. I have examined over fifteen children (not counting the infants) and in no instance have I had any trouble in getting them to cooperate so that I may do my examination." He goes on to attribute his success to a three-pronged approach:

> 1. Most children are "show offs" at heart, so I give them a chance at first and lead them on a little, then in examination they are still trying to "show off" and impress me so that they will do what I ask with perfection if they can.
>
> 2. I try to be very frank and straight forward with them; realizing that a child is really no fool and really likes to be treated somewhat as a grown-up.
>
> 3. I try at first to let them look me over and get used to me before I touch them. A child just doesn't seem to like a stranger until he has sized him up.[10]

Charm (including, no doubt, the appealing grin) was no small part of McGovern's success with children. He would, for instance, incorporate magic tricks like pulling a coin out of thin air behind a child's ear to win attention and cooperation. That his small patients got to keep the coins made the trick all the better. They would wait anxiously to see what he would do next.[11]

At graduation John P. McGovern, MD, recipient of the coveted Borden Prize for student research, was a budding pediatrician ready to apply himself to his calling. The next phase of his career would be his postgraduate internship and residency training.

New Haven and Yale Pediatrics (1945–1946)

McGovern would have liked to start his postgraduate education at Duke, where he had been so successful and was comfortable. But Davison would not have it. He insisted that a student should avoid getting too entrenched in one institution without being exposed to new teachers and their methods in a different environment.[12] Davison certainly wanted his prize student to continue training at Duke, but he felt strongly that at least a year of training outside Durham would be to McGovern's advantage.

McGovern therefore began looking for a pediatric residency program with convenient access to Washington, DC, and his ailing father. It was important to find a rigorous program, one offering the learning opportunity of a lifetime under a strong leader who had, moreover, national recognition. The postgraduate years for a recently graduated medical student—that is, the internship and residency—are critical. During these transitional years, the young physician is no longer tested on exams but must function in the real world of medicine, where the life of the patient is at stake.

McGovern and Davison identified Yale University Medical School's Department of Pediatrics, led by Grover Powers, as the place to be. Using the direct approach of the times, Davison simply picked up the phone, called Powers, and said, "Grover, I've got a young fellow here named Jack McGovern who would make a fine intern for you."[13] McGovern was accepted in principle on the spot and made plans to move to New Haven. He also made an agreement with Davison to return in a year to Duke to complete additional residency training. Clouding this plan was the ongoing war in Europe that could call him up at any time for active duty as a member of the US Army Medical Corps. But this was a service he was prepared to render.

Although it was not without a pang that McGovern left the comfort of his six-year stay in Durham, New Haven and Yale's Department of Pediatrics would prove to be an ideal stopover on his way to his future.

A German physician named Abraham Jacobi (1830–1919) is most often credited as the father of the field McGovern was entering, pediatrics. In fact Jacobi had introduced the term in 1858,[14] half a dozen years after earning his medical degree at the University of Bonn in 1851. Arrested in Berlin while trying to take his state medical exams, Jacobi was convicted of treason and imprisoned for promoting political and social reform as part of the German revolutionary movement.[15] In 1853, with letters of introduction from his friend Karl Marx, he arrived in New York City, where he set up a low-fee medical practice in the Bowery and quickly developed a large following.

In 1861 Jacobi was named professor of childhood diseases at New York Medical College. Later he was given an appointment as clinical professor of diseases of children at Columbia's College of Physicians and Surgeons and taught at Columbia from 1870 to 1902. The appointment established him as the first professor of pediatrics in the United States.[16] Throughout his medical career Jacobi championed children's care. In 1888, along with Sir William Osler and others, he was a guiding force launching the

American Pediatric Society, which he served as its first president. He produced more than two hundred academic publications during his lifetime. Highly respected by his peers, in 1912 he became the first foreign-born president of the American Medical Association. He died on July 10, 1919, at eighty-nine.[17]

No pediatrics department existed at Johns Hopkins when Osler arrived as chief of medicine in 1889. That changed in 1912, the year Jacobi took the reins of the AMA, when Johns Hopkins appointed John Howland as chairman of its newly opened Harriet Lane Home for Invalid Children, which put in place the model pediatrics program of its day. The innovative facility had isolation wings for children with infectious diseases and laboratories for finding treatments for such pediatric scourges as rheumatic fever, polio, and rickets.[18]

With medical degrees from both New York University College (1897) and Cornell University (1899), Howland was legendary in the emerging field of pediatrics; in fact, he was considered by many to be the best pediatrician in the world. He was highly sought after by other universities, and when Harvard made a bid for him, Howland generated newspaper headlines like a sports figure. On May 29, 1921, a *New York Times* headline, if it didn't precisely scream, at least bawled loudly in an oversized font, "Declines Harvard Offer—Dr. John Howland to Remain at Johns Hopkins."[19]

Howland's star faculty member at Johns Hopkins, Edwards A. Park (1877–1969), was also a much sought-after commodity. Park, a 1905 graduate of Columbia's College of Physicians and Surgeons, had a strong background in biochemical research, which he had done in Germany. This was supplemented by nine years of work in Howland's pioneering pediatrics program at Hopkins. Park's background caught the eye of many, and Dean Milton C. Winternitz recruited him as founding chair of the new pediatrics department at Yale. Park arrived in New Haven on July 1, 1921 (the year McGovern was born), and high on his list of priorities at Yale was to recruit his own star associate from Hopkins—another Howland protégé, Grover Powers (1887–1967).[20] In addition to Powers, Park recruited a number of other outstanding faculty who would in time make big names, including Martha Eliot, who went on to lead the nation's Children's Bureau. Eliot was not the only woman on Park's faculty; in fact, four of the eleven outstanding people Park recruited were women—an uncommon testament to his forward thinking and his ability to recognize talent.[21] Along with the strong faculty, Park brought to Yale an integrated approach to the medical care of children that combined rigorous research with strong training programs and community outreach.

Of special interest to Park was study of the cause and treatment of rickets, a disease that was also of particular interest to Howland and was endemic in New Haven.

Only five years after Park started the new pediatrics program at Yale, the untimely and unexpected death of Howland from cirrhosis of the liver on June 20, 1926, while he was visiting clinics in London, brought Park back to Baltimore as Howland's replacement at Johns Hopkins. Grover Powers then advanced to the departmental chair at Yale. Powers proved an outstanding choice. From 1926 to 1951 he built on Park's vision. He trained a generation of the best and brightest in pediatrics, including Jack McGovern, and molded the pediatrics department into one of the most respected in the country. To this day the Powers years are affectionately known in pediatrics circles as the Golden Age of pediatrics at Yale.[22]

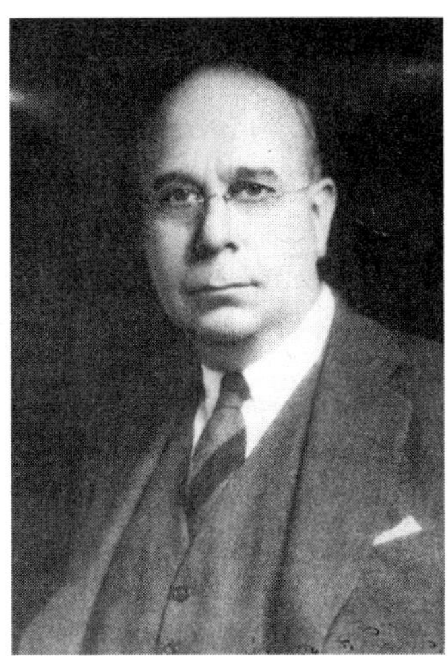

FIGURE 3.1. Grover F. Powers, chairman of pediatrics at Yale.

Howard Pearson, a former chairman of the department (1974–1986), has written extensively on its history. Looking back to those early days, he notes that "Powers became one of the great figures in the American pediatrics of his day, not because of his scientific accomplishments, but because of his unique personality, clinical prowess, and teaching skills. . . . for 25 years he made an indelible impression and left a lasting legacy in American pediatrics."[23]

The year at Yale was a time of professional maturation for McGovern. To begin with, he had the exposure at another school that Davison had recommended to give him perspective and practical experience outside his comfort zone. Through the influence of Park, Yale reinforced McGovern's interest in research and discovery; through the influence of Powers, it reinforced the pull that he had always felt toward the humanistic side of pediatrics. In this roundabout way, from Davison to Howland to Park to Powers, McGovern would never be far from the Oslerian tradition of Duke during his advanced pediatrics training at Yale. Indeed, nothing McGovern did in his medical career would fall far from that tradition of humanistic, patient-centered care, with research and discovery guiding the way to improved patient outcomes.

Moreover, McGovern was forever one of "Grover's Boys," as Yale alumni liked to refer to themselves.[24] His students were fond of Powers, and wary. Before McGovern even arrived in New Haven, one of Powers's assistant residents provided some essential advice: "Never, and I mean never, tell Dr. Powers that something isn't done; tell him that it is being done, and it better be started the minute he leaves."[25]

Powers was a demanding perfectionist for whom the patient was a serious human consideration who came first in every way. Morris Wessel recalled when, as a third-year medical student, he went on his first day of rounds with him. Having entered the room with his small group of students, Powers quickly backed out. Outside the door Wessel queried, "Aren't we going to see the patient?"

"The child is eating his breakfast," Powers replied. "You wouldn't expect me to interrupt his meal, would you?"[26]

One of Powers's pet peeves was his opinion that scientific inquiry was insufficiently incorporated into the training for and practice of medicine. He prided himself that Yale was one of the few medical schools in the country requiring a research thesis for graduation. No doubt McGovern's Borden Prize for best research project in his class was a factor in Powers's good opinion of him.

Powers taught his students to notice the tiniest, subtlest changes in a patient's situation. His powers of observation seemed to rival those of Sherlock Holmes. Alumni of his program marveled years later at Powers's sensitivity to the pain and sufferings of others. He could glance into a patient's room and within seconds list three differences from earlier in the day and four questions that needed asking.[27]

In his final retirement address delivered at Yale in 1951, the aging Powers, now professor emeritus, looked back on his years at Yale and the many outstanding students he had trained, and summarized what the calling of medicine was all about:

> Some years ago an alumnus of this school and its department of pediatrics became chief resident in a large university hospital not too far distant. In the course of time I received a letter from a friend who is chief of the pediatric service in that hospital. I sent the letter to the mother of the young doctor so I cannot quote it exactly, but the message it carried was as follows:
>
> I thought you would like to have me tell you of an experience I had the other night with Dr. Blank. I was called to the hospital at midnight by another member of the house staff to see a private patient. As I passed the public ward I saw Dr. Blank working at the bedside of a sick baby. I happened to know it was his night off duty and I chastised him gently for staying around. I thought you would like to know his comment—where I come from you do not leave the ward when you are needed to care for a sick patient.[28]

Who can say if "Dr. Blank" was Jack McGovern and the mother was Lottie Brown McGovern? Regardless, this was the caliber of physician—and man—a Grover's Boy was trained to be. And McGovern measured up to Powers's expectations on all counts.

Powers believed that medicine should deal not just with the diseases of the body but also with those of the mind and spirit: "It is our responsibility," he wrote, "to understand the culturally deprived, the emotionally disturbed, the mentally retarded." Working with the State of Connecticut, he created the Southbury Training School, an enlightened and humane facility that served developmentally disabled children and was headed by one of Powers's leading faculty, Herman Yannet.[29]

It was here that McGovern would spend a rotation of seven weeks addressing the medical needs of such children, but not before contracting a severe case of infectious mononucleosis that gave him a memorable experience of being a patient. It cost him six long weeks of convalescence that he could ill afford. Concerned letters from his parents following this illness would commonly end with "Get your rest," "Don't try to go too fast,"[30] "Keep on the beam,"[31] and "Don't work too hard."[32] They were well acquainted with the fact that their son did not know how to slow down and rest. Idleness was anathema to him. Years later McGovern would recall that being a patient had been exceedingly unpleasant.[33] Being confined to a bed while he wanted fervently to be up and about his business was torture.

However, he also learned a happier lesson from being confined, namely, that he very much liked the corn fritters served at the Yale-New Haven Hospital dining room; and they sharpened his taste for a good dose of hot Tabasco sauce from Louisiana. Other residents recalled that after the experience, McGovern always had a small bottle of Tabasco sauce buried deep in the pocket of his white coat to "fix the fritters."[34]

Having overcome his bout with mono, McGovern joined Yannet at the Southbury Training School and demonstrated a renewed love of his work. If anything, he seemed to be recharged by his illness. In Yannet's telling,

> We were a small medical group at that time; but what we lacked in numbers we made up in enthusiasm. And I do remember that John, always pleasant and smiling, made a significant contribution to that enthusiasm. My cottage and ward rounds with him every morning made my days a pleasure. Soon after his arrival, he indicated a desire to study in depth some basic medical problem that involved an appreciable number of our patients. I suggested a study of a small group of cerebral palsy patients whose motor disabilities, unlike so many others, were asymmetrical. Perhaps, I added, such a study might throw some light on the relative importance of certain etiologies as related to the type and degree of the palsied condition. He spent most of his free time pursuing this problem, and before he left, he had put together the material to serve as the basis for the first contribution to the medical literature. The article was published in early 1947 and was well received. Of the more than 300 to 400 interns and residents that have participated in the New Haven rotation program, I can count on the fingers of one hand those who carried out to completion such medical studies. It was probably an omen of his future progress and subsequent achievement.[35]

Department chair Grover Powers took notice of the impressive work ethic and follow-through that separated McGovern from many others. The year went quickly. Despite an offer from Powers to stay on at Yale for a second year, McGovern wanted to go back to Duke as planned. He politely declined Yale.

But military duty called, and Davison provided the notice on November 16, 1945:"The rumor I mentioned in my letter of October 8 that all the Army interns will be called to active duty and that no deferments for assistant residencies will be allowed has just been made official. According to the last directive, you will be called to active duty on July 1, 1946. I regret more than I can tell you that you will not be with us the coming year but am looking forward to your returning after your Army service. I hope."[36]

Wheelchairs and Chairoteers (1946–1948)

Initially assigned to the Oteen Veterans Administration Hospital near Ashville, North Carolina, McGovern, a young captain in the Army Medical Corps, was soon transferred to a larger veterans' facility, McGuire General Hospital in Richmond, Virginia. This was a period of continued decline in McGovern's father's health, and the transfer to Richmond placed him within a hundred miles of his parents, no doubt providing them and him alike a greater peace of mind.

At age twenty-seven, it was clear to McGovern that his father, at fifty-five, was succumbing to tuberculosis and hepatitis. McGovern summarized the situation to Davison: "I had just returned from Braddock Heights where I had spent several days helping Mother take care of Dad. Ten days ago he came down with the prodromal symptoms of homologous serum hepatitis followed in four days by severe jaundice then progressive loss of contact and two days ago complete coma."[37]

Months earlier his father had undergone a procedure known as thoracoplasty, which entailed removing six to eight ribs and collapsing the pleural cavity—a painful course of action then used as a last resort for gravely ill tuberculosis patients. The procedure was replaced a decade later in the late 1950s by new anti-tuberculosis drugs.[38]

Jack McGovern had always been sensitive to the delicate equilibrium that defines health in terms of physical, mental, and social well-being.[39] That understanding would be a great asset in his new assignment at the McGuire General Hospital in Richmond. Freshly arrived there, he was assigned to the Department of Physical Medicine and Rehabilitation, where he was appointed assistant director of the Physical Medicine Service. His new position placed him in charge of the paraplegic service, which

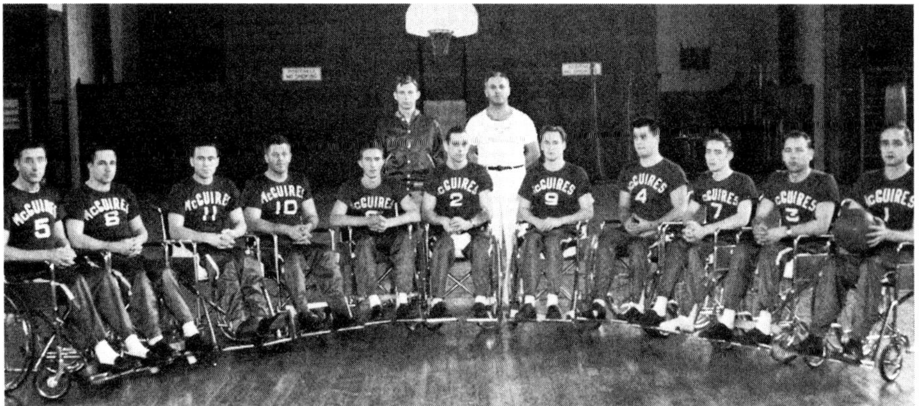

FIGURE 3.2. McGovern (in white) with his Chairoteers basketball team.

cared for more than 150 young veterans—all, to the man, paraplegics with dreams of bright futures dashed by the ugliest side of World War II, which had just ended with the surrender of Japan less than a year before.

The medical corps struggled to address the growing numbers of young soldiers returning in wheelchairs. McGovern could see in his patients' eyes their misery at being trapped inside their bodies—mentally alert, full of unchanneled energy, and frustrated. The solution, he surmised, might be found in channeling their frustration constructively. McGovern would not accept the loss of physical capabilities as the loss of the whole person.

If health is a delicate balance of physical, mental, and social well-being, then having two of the three seemed to McGovern a good start for overcoming what must have looked to these soldiers like impossible odds. Across the country veterans' hospitals were searching for an outlet for these young men who were struggling to adapt to their new norm of life in a wheelchair. Organized sports such as ping-pong, bowling, swimming, water polo, and basketball were all explored as interventions for wheelchair-bound veterans.

McGovern seized on the idea of organized basketball. Within months of his arrival, his enthusiasm and energy proved just what his paraplegic patients needed to build a strong new sense of common identity and camaraderie. They formed a basketball team on wheels known as the Chairoteers and soon were playing teams from other VA hospitals including Boston,

Chicago, Memphis, and New York. From these early VA teams, wheelchair basketball would develop into the sport we know today.

"Our boys always won against fine college and university teams, who were no match when having to play in wheelchairs and by our rules," recalled McGovern some years later.[40] Those who worked with McGovern in the years ahead found special meaning in this statement, because he always played to win, and anytime he could write the rules, and practice to perfection—competition, beware!

During this period he also made time to moonlight by helping two local pediatricians with their practices. One of them, Edwin Kendig, had returned from the war and a bout with pulmonary tuberculosis to find his solo practice booming with more patients than he could handle. "From my standpoint," he wrote, "Jack was a godsend, and for Jack it was his first experience in clinical pediatric practice.... That Jack would become prominent in the field of allergy and immunology never crossed my mind. It was easy to see, however, that he would be successful, whatever his chosen endeavor."[41]

From this opportunity came McGovern's first experience in private practice, the idea of which would evolve over time in his own career planning as he weighed a full-time academic career against the independence of operating his own clinic. And there was the even better possibility of owning a private practice and holding academic appointments in the medical departments of local universities.

McGovern found time to take on several research projects during his army assignment in Richmond, and one of these in particular broadened his medical interests beyond pediatrics. By happenstance, a friend who was a dentist developed a numbness and swelling of the tongue and upper lip after eating ice cream. When McGovern questioned him, he reported other adverse reactions to cold exposure as well.[42] McGovern then researched cold urticaria (a condition now recognized as a form of hives or red welts initiated by a histamine reaction) and managed his friend's allergic reaction successfully, which, in turn, led to his first published paper in the *Journal of Allergy*.[43]

Never far from his paraplegic patients and the Chairoteers, whose winning record was the talk of the VA system, he understood that self-help information was needed. He wrote guides and aids for his patients in his spare time—an important form of patient education that he continued throughout his career—assuring that his patients always left his care with practical information in writing to share with family and put to use.[44]

As Mac McGovern's health continued to decline, a letter arrived addressed to him from a patient in Ward 17-E, Bed 13, of McGuire General Hospital—a carefully typed and formatted letter that must have brought a moment of pleasure to the ailing surgeon, whose pleasures now were few; he lived his professional life through the successes of his son.

> *March 31, 1947*
> *Dear Doctor McGovern:*
>
> *The other day I happened into the snack bar of this great hospital. There I saw a young doctor whose face was very familiar. He turned out to be Dr. John McGovern, assistant chief, Physical Medicine, your son, to whom I had taught typewriting some ten or eleven years ago in Woodrow Wilson High School. . . .*
>
> *He was friendly, charming and gracious to his old school teacher. He has been so successful, and has given definite promise of doing outstanding research work and studies. Only today I found him studying statistics for the purpose of working out correlations needed in some studies he had made using children and mice.*
>
> *He is extremely popular here not only with the staff but with the patients as well. Both respect him for his understanding and high technical skill. In treating the disease he has not forgotten to treat the patient.*
>
> *You have every right to be extremely happy and proud because there is no greater achievement than giving to society for its service an educated, competent and successful citizen of this democracy of ours. . . .*
>
> *Sincerely[,]*
> *Joseph L. Kochka*[45]

Such a letter must have warmed the cockles of Mac's heart.

When McGovern completed his military duty, he had gained much practical experience in pediatrics, explored the advantages and disadvantages of working in private practice, furthered his own research interests, and made a difference for his paraplegic patients and other veterans throughout the hospital. The progress of his paraplegic patients at McGuire General Hospital, and the physical, mental, and social benefits of wheelchair basketball, were not lost on the Department of Veterans Affairs. In 1980 the VA formally established a Recreation Therapy Service.[46] Wheelchair sports as a therapeutic tool for treating veterans with disabilities is today a highly organized, international program.[47]

Home Again and Paris-Bound (1948–1949)

True his word, Dean Davison brought McGovern back to Durham to continue his residency training in pediatrics. It was July of 1948. McGovern would be appointed one of two assistant residents to the chief resident in pediatrics and would report to the Howland Pediatric Ward, now overflowing with patients as a result of the country's post-war polio epidemic.

Returning to Duke and following Davison on rounds was a comfortable and much anticipated transition for McGovern. He reunited with his former roommate, Ziggy, now a Duke pediatrics resident, and the two teamed up on a research project resulting in a presentation at the meeting of the American Federation for Clinical Research in New Orleans. It would be McGovern's first paper presentation and his first trip to the Big Easy—a foreshadowing of hundreds of presentations at professional societies in years to come, and the first trip to a city he would one day call home as a faculty member at Tulane University School of Medicine (1954–1956).

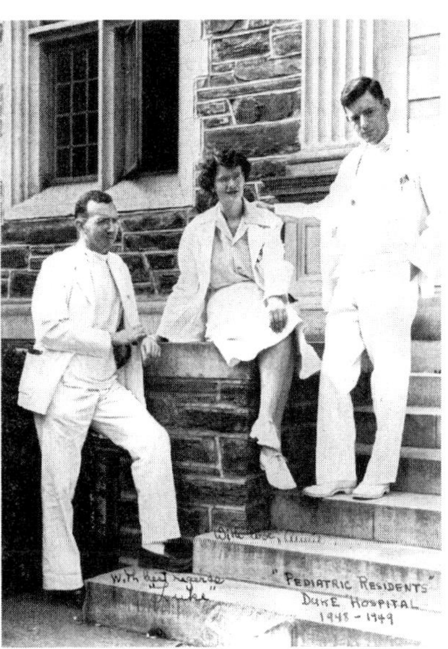

FIGURE 3.3. McGovern (right) as a pediatric resident at Duke Hospital in 1949. With Harry B. "Luke" O'Rear and Annie Bestebreurtje.

James Caddy, another Duke resident, remembered that when McGovern returned to Duke from the service, he weighed about 120 pounds and was "always carrying reference books and was always one step ahead of the pack of residents and interns and one step behind Dean Davison. Jack always seemed to be interested in how and why something worked or didn't work and was always quoting literature that he read so thoroughly and was even then contributing to."[48]

In a somewhat unexpected move, Davison surprised McGovern during his residency by offering him a fellowship, including a travel scholarship, to study at Guy's Hospital in London and the Hôpital des Enfants-Malades in Paris during the spring and early summer of 1949. Davison understood by now that McGovern was extraordinary, not only a Borden Prize-caliber researcher but a physician of Oslerian qualities who in short order had impressed the very best at Yale and the powers throughout the Veterans Administration as well. As Osler and Davison had been, McGovern was anxious to see for himself the bigger picture of medicine through a sojourn to London and Paris, where tradition and medical history are measured in centuries, not decades.

He followed in the footsteps of many other physicians from North America whose education was not considered complete until they had seen the great institutions and traditions of Europe. Armed with letters of introduction from Davison to the pediatrics chiefs at hospitals throughout Paris and London, McGovern was about to leave the United States on his first trip abroad.

He was ready, but how would he get there on his tight budget with minimal travel expense? For suggestions he turned to his cousin Helen Hayes in New York. She replied:

November 27, 1948
Dear Jack,
That's a very exciting prospect—your going to London to study. I'm sure you'll enjoy your experience there as I did mine.
Will you send me two short typewritten letters explaining about your prospects—going to London to study, that you wish to work your way over, etc. I will find someone in the Cunard Line and the United States Line to send each letter with a note of my own, and will see if there's some way of getting you on one of the ships. You might add what post you think you would best fit.
Love to the family,
As always,
Helen[49]

McGovern was soon onboard the SS *America* and off to London with a second stop in Paris. Owned by the United States Lines, the 723-foot ship had been completed in 1940 by the Newport News Shipbuilding and Drydock Company in Virginia and outfitted for 1,202 passengers and 643 crew.[50] Helen's contacts had paid off, as McGovern was given first-class status with minimal demands on his medical expertise. During World War II the ship had been in service as the USS *West Point,* painted in camouflage gray and capable of carrying more than seven thousand troops. In 1941, two Nazi spies had joined her crew to obtain information about the movement of ships and military defense preparations at the Panama Canal. The Duquesne spy ring was soon uncovered by the FBI and involved thirty-one German agents. Their conviction was the largest espionage conviction in US history at the time.[51] By 1946 the ship was once again the SS *America* and was considered by many in these pre-Queen Mary days of the Cunard Line as the most beautifully decorated liner to fly the American flag.[52]

McGovern's twelve-week trip had both backwards and forwards significance. When the SS *America* left New York Harbor on March 18, 1949, it was carrying McGovern to the great hospitals of London and Paris, where he would meet and work with physicians and scientists whose value to his career he could hardly have anticipated. At the same time, the ship was parting waters that had brought McGovern's great grandfather Philip McGovern to America as he fled the Irish Famine a century earlier. And it was carrying McGovern to Guy's Hospital in London, the same first stop Osler had made upon leaving McGill for Europe in 1872.[53] Thus McGovern was carrying on a tradition of studying at Guy's that would not have been lost on Wilburt Davison.

The hospital was founded in 1721 by Thomas Guy, who made his fortune publishing unlicensed Bibles. Guy was associated with the South Sea Company that had been granted a monopoly for British trade with South America and had made some insider investors rich and many more flat broke after the bubble burst and the company failed in 1720. Guy's insider fortune, however, was put to good use, as he funded the creation of Guy's Hospital to treat "incurables" discharged from St. Thomas Hospital.[54]

Osler's trip had been made possible by his older brother Edmund, a highly successful Canadian banker who advanced Osler $1000 (a very large sum in today's money) to fund his time abroad.[55] McGovern's trip was funded by a study grant that Davison found to provide financial assistance for his mentee. Almost as important as the funding support were Davison's highly entertaining stories of his own exploits through Europe during and after his Oxford days with Osler, which heightened McGovern's anticipation of his coming adventure.

As a student of Osler's, Davison had built his career, even his own medical school, around the network of connections he had established and experiences he had had during his years at Oxford (1913–1916) and in subsequent military service with the American Expeditionary Force (1917–1919). His own experiences during World War I had taken him to hospitals and clinics throughout Europe, providing him a global perspective on health care that he could have acquired no other way. Moreover, Osler and Nobel laureate Sir Charles Sherrington (a pioneer in neurophysiology) had given Davison his own letters of introduction, and these had proven invaluable. One favorite story of Davison's that McGovern loved to retell was about a letter of introduction Osler had provided Davison and fellow Rhodes scholar Wilder Penfield as an entrée to visit the renowned London surgeon Sir Arbuthnot Lane, 1st Baronet, in his clinic at Guy's Hospital.

Early in the visit Davison differed with his host regarding whether the steel plates Lane was using to fix a patient's broken leg were actually superior to the autogenous bone grafts touted by the American Fred F. Albee. Albee had claimed the plates would bend and could not compare to bone grafts.

Davison, when challenged by Lane to bend one of the steel plates with his bare hands, did just that. "After all," he commented later, "I had been rowing for six years and had fairly strong hands and shoulders. Sir Arbuthnot's astonished face as I handed him the bent plate was purple." Lane asked for Davison's name. "I handed him Osler's note of introduction, and Sir Arbuthnot's belligerent manner immediately changed. He spent the rest of the day with Penfield and me trying to atone for his rudeness, took us all over Guy's Hospital and drove us to the American Embassy in his car."[56]

Now McGovern himself was on his way to see these places in London and Paris that he had heard so much about. On the trip over, he was already learning firsthand that having connections and means can smooth the journey ahead. On March 21, 1949, he wrote his parents:

> This is the first opportunity for a letter to be sent from the ship. . . . I was extremely fortunate in being seated at the Captain's table which is more

> of an honor than I expected aboard ship. . . . There are in all eight at our table, all very nice folks. A Mr. and Mrs. Young en route to London (He is Pres. of the Rubber Importers) have invited me to stay in their Suite in London at the Savoy the night we arrive there. That will give me time to call the doctors and get oriented. It sure is good that I brought my tux as I wear it every night to dinner. Tonight is the Captain's dinner and we have Champagne and many festivities.
>
> The food is better than even New Orleans cuisine. I have had steak or roast beef about every night. Oysters, crepes suzette, shrimp and lobster salads. You can not imagine what wonderful food. I don't think that I'll get a pot belly though.[57]

But more important to McGovern than day-to-day social experiences was the overall sense of being a part of historical seats of medical discovery. It is one thing to know the European heroes of medical history like Pasteur, Lister, Koch, the great French surgeon Paré. It is another to walk the corridors they walked, to see the tradition and style of the great hospitals in action, and to lay eyes on the very laboratories and surgical suites from which great European medical discoveries emerged.

In the 1830s American doctors went to Paris to study because American medical schools were inadequate. Paris and its famous Ecole de Médecine were then a mecca for physicians like Oliver Wendell Homes (1809–1894), father of Supreme Court Justice Oliver Wendell Holmes (1841–1935), who wanted to train with the best at the world's leading center of medicine. It has been said that in the mid-1800s the population of medical Paris equaled that of a small city and included every variety of humankind and virtually every known ailment and affliction.[58] America offered nothing like what Paris offered. It would be 1910 before Abraham Flexner would release his transforming report on the need of American and Canadian medical schools to reform or close their doors.[59]

Unlike the education of American medical students in Paris a century before, McGovern's education during the mid-1940s was considered the world standard, despite lacking the international and historical perspective that Davison knew would round out his prize student's edges. McGovern's letters home during these twelve weeks show him excited, busy, and grateful for the rare chance he has happened into. He is staying with the Firths on Streatham Common and eager to be pleased:

> Their house is lovely and [Mrs. Firth] treats me just as nice as you could imagine. We have breakfast each A.M. at 8 and I will be at the hospital at 8:45 each day. Start regularly at Guy's tomorrow. Will stay there about 3 weeks and then move on to St. Bartholomews. I am a lucky young man to have this opportunity. I assure you and know that these 2½ months will mean more to me than any comparable length of time in my life. Not only just from the medical point of view but to live with these people broadens one's outlook considerably. There are so many things that I have learned already that I can't adequately begin to tell them.[60]

Letters, carefully dated, arrived weekly from McGovern describing his impressions of London and Paris for his parents, who had never traveled abroad and now did so vicariously through their son's experiences. On April 3, 1949, he writes, "I have now been in London 10 days. It has been 10 days filled with more interesting and satisfactory experiences for me. . . . It would have been difficult for me to have imagined better circumstances to have fallen into than those of the moment."[61] Armed with introductions from Davison, McGovern made the rounds of faculty and wards at Guys. He quickly acclimated to the pace and style of British medicine—including sunning and casual lunch on the hospital's lawn with his newfound colleagues.

Particularly agreeable to McGovern were the special lectures, tours by senior faculty of their research laboratories, and morning rounds with patients assigned to him during his visit. All were chronicled in his letters home. "My good fortune in making such wonderful contacts is amazing indeed," he wrote.

When he crossed the English Channel and arrived in Paris on the night of May 18, he immediately wrote home, "It was rather sad leaving London and all of my new found friends there. . . . Now what about Paris? Too early to say much yet but it looks like it's all it's cracked up to be"[62] Within days he was regaling his parents with the sights of the great city and his adventures in it despite the handicap of not speaking French. The Louvre, the Eiffel Tower, the Palais Garnier (where he attended *La Traviata*), the Arche de Triomphe, and especially Versailles made a strong impression on him and found their place in his letters.

For Lottie, known for her love of cooking, he talked about the bargain French cuisine in which he indulged: "I had a wonderful steak dinner with French salad and Vin Rouge, plus French pastry for desert for only

510 francs [about $1.50)."[63] At restaurants McGovern's frugal side always seemed to be on high alert; he kept a guarded vigilance over his pocketbook that might have made the notoriously thrifty Osler himself smile. He was convinced that the French were on a mission to separate him from his money: "No matter where you go the French cheat you—they can add 10 francs on to each thing faster than an adding machine can count. I always go to the same café where I am now known as 'le bon monsieur, le bon docteur' and am consequently cheated a little less than the usual amount."[64] McGovern's penny-wise habits persisted into later years even as his personal wealth soared into the millions. He would forever fret over any discrepancy, whether it involved a multimillion-dollar real estate deal or change from a dollar.

Other discoveries captured the young American bachelor's attention—"The French women are all that is said of them particularly the Parisians. They really dress and look beautiful."[65] Soon he is looking forward to a party at which he will meet two French girlfriends of a friend: "That could be good fun for believe me, everything that is said about French girls is true."[66]

McGovern was already a prodigious collector of rare medical books and smitten with a special interest in medical medallions (highly collectable and frequently rare coin-sized medallions often struck in bronze or silver to commemorate famous physicians or events in medical history).[67] Paris proved to be a bonanza for his collecting instincts, just as it had been for Osler, Cushing, Davison, and so many others before them who had prowled the bookshops to fill their libraries and biblio addictions. "I have, as in London, spent many hours walking thru the avenues and in and out of the many antique and bookstores," he writes to his parents on May 28. "Have added many finds to my growing medical medallion collection and think that my collection has almost reached the proportion where it would be worth exhibiting. It has been a growing hobby with me and far more educational and worthwhile than ever planned. You know that I am a collector by nature."[68]

While his letters home overflowed with the sights of Paris, his primary mission was to gain experience and attend patients at the Hôpital des Enfants-Malades in Paris. This too he accomplished. The hospital was founded in 1802 by Paris's General Hospices Council "for the children of both sexes under the age of fifteen years" and is considered the first pediatric hospital in the Western world.[69] Located adjacent to it on the Rue de Sèvres is Paris's famous Necker Hospital, founded in 1778 and devoted to medicine and surgery in adults. In 1920, the year before McGovern's birth, the two hospitals merged. The Necker Hospital is most famously known as the hospital where French physician Laennec invented the stethoscope in 1816.[70]

The opportunity to attend patients and walk the halls of the Hôpital des Enfants-Malades was a rite of passage, a capstone on McGovern's pediatrics training. Each day he met new faculty and attended rounds, acquiring a sound appreciation for the French system of health-care delivery. Additionally, his newfound appreciation for French people and their culture would stay with him a lifetime. Years later he would conduct research with French colleagues, even receive a national commendation and appointment from President François Mitterand to the French National Order of Merit for his work with French scientists in the field of chronobiology,[71] the study of our inherent biological clocks and their relationship to health and illness.

McGovern returned to Duke in the summer of 1949 a more independent man, more self-assured, and possessed of a renewed sense of his destiny. His letters home suggest greater self-confidence. In many ways his education in Europe signaled a metamorphosis from son and student to physician and scholar. From here on he would advise and watch over his parents rather than seek their guidance.

Now the son was counseling both parents as he concluded his final letter home from Paris, which began with a word of assurance for his mother. "Your 'nervousness' is probably due most to the strain of renting the house and now that it is over you will become your good old self again."[72] Later, in the same letter, McGovern (a smoker himself who would quit cold turkey in 1966) provided encouragement and medical advice for his ailing father: "I believe that smoking has a really deleterious effect on T.B. in many ways. . . . I think that it also destroys a certain amount of general sense of well-being and desire to do all possible to affect cure. Obviously you really think so too or you wouldn't have exerted the tremendous will-power necessary to stop smoking. I myself know how hard it is and I'm not the confirmed smoker that you were."[73]

At the conclusion of his trip abroad McGovern had seen through his own eyes the great medical institutions that had once made such profound impressions on his mentors. He had also measured himself against others in medicine an ocean away. And his desire to build a library of rare books and preserve medical history had crystallized. He had long been familiar with an observation of Osler's that Davison had preached to his Duke students for years: "To study the phenomena of disease without books is to sail an uncharted sea, while to study books without patients is not to go to sea at all."[74] He left Europe prepared to act on that observation—perhaps because Europe had made him more aware of the real possibility of actually getting the kinds of books he wanted. Quite simply, he was a butterfly out of pupae and ready to take flight.

George Washington University and Markel Scholar (1949–1950)

In July of 1949, his postgraduate training and his study abroad complete, McGovern returned to Washington, DC, to assume his first faculty position, as an associate in pediatrics (he was shortly promoted to assistant professor) at George Washington School of Medicine and chief of the George Washington University Pediatrics Division at District of Columbia General Hospital. It was the first of seventeen professorships that he would hold at fifteen universities during his professional life.

In 1821 President James Monroe first approved the congressional charter that established Columbian College in the District of Columbia, later known as George Washington School of Medicine. The first commencement two years later was a great source of civic pride and was attended by such dignitaries as President Monroe, Henry Clay, John C. Calhoun, and the great French patriot who had fought with George Washington in the American Revolution, the Marquis de Lafayette. By the end of the Civil War, Columbian College was renamed Columbian University and moved downtown to 15th and H Streets. In 1904 it was renamed a second time as George Washington University in honor of the first US president; and in 1912 it was relocated to the DC neighborhood of Foggy Bottom.[75] In more contemporary times it is remembered as the emergency room credited with saving the life of President Ronald Reagan following an attempted assassination at the Washington Hilton Hotel on March 30, 1981.[76]

In July 1949, three decades before President Reagan was rushed to George Washington with a bullet in his lung, McGovern had arrived there to launch his academic career as a newly appointed faculty member. While Davison had made more than one offer to his prize student for a faculty appointment at Duke, McGovern needed to remain close to his parents;

his father's life was drawing to a close. The opportunity to join the faculty of George Washington Hospital offered both proximity to his family and a chance to prove himself the triple hitter in medicine that he would rapidly become as physician, teacher, and researcher.

For starters, he would face a tough crowd of second-year students, the class of 1952. With a median age of twenty-six, they were World War II veterans almost to the man. All were in a hurry, with little time or interest in idle talk. They filled the medical school's amphitheater, which was designed in the classic tradition, narrow toward the lecturer's dais and fanning steeply up thirty-odd rows. In the words of Dorris Merritt, one of the few female fellows on the faculty, McGovern would be tested by a very difficult crowd:

> They knew what they were there for and poor teaching was not on the list. One instructor had actually been booed to the point of such personal demoralization that he resigned at mid-year. Into this receptive atmosphere strode John P. McGovern. . . . [He] approached that cynical class precisely as if we were the collective two-year-old he was teaching us to examine. He offered his priceless gifts of enthusiasm, devotion to his specialty, and a total commitment to the standards of clinical excellence coupled with regard for the history of medicine. . . . Nor was it coincidental that, in a class where only three graduates became full-time members of a medical school faculty, two of them selected pediatrics.[77]

Davison's prize student hit the ground running in the classroom, clinics, and research labs of George Washington University. Whether in the amphitheatre or one of the affiliated hospitals, such as Gallinger Municipal, where he maintained a small unairconditioned office (common for the time),[78] his broad grin, coupled with confidence and high-octane energy, won over the students in his charge. On all fronts faculty and students alike described him as dedicated, restless, and driven. That love of medicine he had written home about during his student days at Duke now commanded all his energies and grabbed the attention of everyone who crossed his path.

In only a year he was elected to membership in the Smith-Reed-Russell Society honor society, which later became a chapter of Alpha Omega Alpha.[79] Students, self-described as a "raucous, cynical class,"[80] had voted him outstanding teacher of the year and sought him out for advice and additional opportunities to follow him in clinic. He was, for anyone half paying attention, a man on the rise.

McGovern's students would remember years later the influence he had on their early training both at the bedside of young patients and in the lecture hall as he regaled them with stories about Davison and Osler. In the clinics he was known for his practice of magic and sleight of hand to put his young patients at ease.[81] One second-year medical student, Donald Fernbach, recalls the young professor's impact on him, which guided his career into the field of pediatrics:

> There is no doubt that most of my classmates will similarly remember Jack as a teacher, because he was one of those rare student stimulators—an inspirational enthusiastic teacher who could find and instill interest in all sorts of clinical circumstances. One day he spent a full hour showing our group how to approach a crying, apprehensive 15-month-old baby. When the demonstration concluded, the child had been thoroughly seduced to complete acquiescence, and each of us was able to examine the then calm, curious little creature who seemed almost disappointed when we finally moved on.[82]

Fellow faculty members were equally impressed. While McGovern had once told his father that a million dollars wouldn't get him interested in a career as a psychiatrist, his training and travels had opened his mind, and fellow faculty like Reginald Lourie were quick to diagnose his formula for success:

> By the time I met Jack McGovern at the Children's Hospital in Washington, DC, he had already developed the ability to fly, having nested with and absorbed large amounts of learning from the great pediatric teachers such as Wilburt Davison at Duke and Grover Powers at Yale, who had flown very high themselves. He had also discovered that the teachers of the past, such as Osler, had left him much to add to his style of flying. Then, when Jack found the newly established pediatric psychiatry program at Children's Hospital, he was well prepared to include this relatively new dimension in his armamentarium. It then became apparent that his greatest talent was the ability to integrate the information from a variety of fields and fly with these syntheses into new directions. This he has

done with pediatrics, allergy, the behavioral sciences, and history, all held together by his own innate contribution, common sense and energy.[83]

The energy McGovern demonstrated in the clinics and classroom was matched by the strength of his attraction to research. His interests in allergies and immunology were emerging. While directing George Washington's clinical clerkship program for the Department of Pediatrics, he met Robert A. Cooke and immediately grew interested in Cooke's successful effort to establish the first allergy clinic for the District of Columbia General Hospital, which served low-income patients. McGovern took notice and studied how an allergy clinic is built from the ground up, thus acquiring insights he would use himself in the future.

An early research project involved the Nickerson-Kveim intracutaneous test for sarcoidosis in children, a disease in which abnormal collections of chronic inflammatory cells, granulomas, form as nodules in multiple organ sites, especially the lungs, where scarring or infection may lead to respiratory failure. This systemic immune system disorder has been implicated (not without controversy) as a health concern among rescue workers and survivors of the 9/11 World Trade Center collapse. More recently the comic Bernie Mac, along with football great Reggie White, have both died of sarcoidosis-related illnesses.

In McGovern's time, very little was known about the disease in children. Initially he wanted to conduct a comprehensive literature review of every reported case of sarcoidosis in children at the time—not just in the United States, but worldwide. His research assistant at the time, Doris Merritt, had her doubts: "When I mentioned a knowledge of Polish, Hungarian, and Russian was hardly at the tip of my tongue, he wasn't the least perturbed. After all, he asked, what were language dictionaries for? . . . The product of that search resulted in what is still the world's most comprehensive review of the sarcoidosis literature, and a shoe box of some 1,000 well-verified reference cards was deposited in the AFML, now in the National Library of Medicine."[84]

McGovern's literature review, *Bibliography on Sarcoidosis (1876–1963)*, would be published by the Public Health Service in 1965 and was the first of twenty-six medically related books he would produce during his career.

"What a great, multi-feathered bird he has become, with at least four wings!," proclaimed senior faculty member Reginald Lourie. Lourie, with his prestigious distinction of having been named a Markle Scholar, was soon consulted by the school's chairman of pediatrics, Preston McClendon, to consider nominating their young star faculty member for the same honor.[85]

John Markle (1858–1933) was a mining engineer and businessman who had made a fortune after he built the Jeddo drainage tunnel to reclaim Pennsylvania's coal mines, which had been inundated by floods in 1886. With an initial investment of $3 million (later increased to $15 million), he established a foundation at the death of his wife Mary Estelle Robinson (1863–1927).[86] In 1946 John Russell, formerly with the Carnegie Corporation in New York, became the foundation's director and launched the Markle Scholar Program.[87] Only twenty-five Markle Scholars were chosen each year, and a medical school could only nominate one candidate. The prize included financial assistance for five years, to encourage the best and brightest to continue in academic medicine and research rather than leave teaching and discovery for private practice. More important for the young recipient was the prestige and notice among peers that the award guaranteed. It was recognition that would last throughout a career.

During the program's twenty-two year history (1947–1969), only 506 Markle Scholars were chosen, representing ninety medical schools in the United States and Canada,[88] and many of them would become physician/scientists like McGovern who would make international names for themselves—all launched by early Markle Scholar recognition.[89] McGovern was chosen a Markle in 1951. The distinction added to his academic pedigree and his grant-getting abilities.

While Mac McGovern would never recover from his illness to return to his career as a surgeon, he did witness his son's impressive rise as a physician of note and took great pride in it. He died on July 28, 1951, in Washington's Mount Alto Veteran's Hospital. The following day the *New York Times* chronicled his death with a headline, "Francis McGovern, Physician, Is Dead: Ex-Head of Garfield Hospital in Washington Had Been an Advisor to Selective Service."[90] McGovern, the collector, clipped the article and added it to his personal scrapbook of cherished memories.

The grieving son, the bird with four wings, was now beating the sides of his academic cage at George Washington University. During this difficult period he threw himself headlong into his work. Accolades kept coming. He received his first research grants, which made headlines in local newspapers.[91] He received congratulatory notes from colleagues for papers published, was invited to present papers at professional meetings throughout the country, was elected to membership in professional organizations, and found time to pass his boards in pediatrics without missing a beat.

Also during this period Wilburt Davison nominated him for membership in the Cosmos Club, an exclusive club founded in Washington, DC, in 1878 for men distinguished in science, literature, the arts, and public service. For many years McGovern would be the youngest elected member of that exclusive organization. Its ranks have included several US presidents, more than thirty Noble Prize winners, over fifty Pulitzer Prize winners, forty five recipients of the Presidential Medal of Freedom, and a long list of Supreme Court justices. By 1988 members would accept nominations for women in the Cosmos Club. One of the first nominated and elected was McGovern's cousin, Helen Hayes.

Despite his outstanding reputation, even talk of a promotion to associate professor by his department chair, McGovern "was finding GWU's administrative red tape frustrating," recalled Hazel Chumley, his part-time secretary.[92] With limited time and minimal research space, he was already consulting with Davison, who by now was both academic role model and father figure, about his concerns that the university's commitment to support him with time and laboratory space was inadequate and limiting his potential.

But leaving George Washington University, McGovern feared, might jeopardize his five-year Markel funding status. In May of 1952 he told Davison that he had seen the director of the Markel Scholarship program in New York, John Russell, and that "he really understands the basic difficulties here in DC and at the G. W. Medical School."[93]

While because of his father's illness McGovern had declined Davison's repeated requests to return to Duke as a resident, his situation was now different as he sought the best fit for his faculty trajectory. He was seriously looking for greener pastures, something new that would provide the room to grow professionally and make a name for himself independent of Davison and Duke. Alabama was a possibility worth looking into, but, he wrote Davison, "in the meantime, I'll keep sawing wood here."[94] Yet what was most on his mind remained where he should move. In addition to Duke, Davison suggested opportunities in Florida and even tested his former student's interest in pediatric psychiatry.[95]

One opportunity offered by Davison caught McGovern's attention just as George Washington was considering a new promotion for him. It was a promotion that he feared would mean even more administrative responsibilities at the cost of his clinical, teaching, and research interests. What he actually wanted was a more balanced environment, like the one he had enjoyed at Yale under Grover Powers—in a program that emphasized both clinical care and research, with the administrative support to accommodate both. Davison understood and came to the rescue. In a letter dated July 9, 1952 he wrote McGovern: "Ralph Platou, Professor of Pediatrics at Tulane, told me that he was looking for someone with your qualifications and I suggested that he write to you. From all accounts that is a splendid opportunity there. Roger Bost is working in Dr. Platou's clinic and also at the Ochsner Clinic. He seemed very enthusiastic. If Ralph writes you, I should look into it. Why not write him if you are interested?"[96]

McGovern followed up on the suggestion during the coming year as his work continued to pile on at George Washington. But among a sea of letters pouring in during this time congratulating him on an assortment of accomplishments, one stands out as very different—a sign, perhaps, of the stresses that this crossroad in the course of his career inflicted. Although McGovern was a paragon of professionalism in the hospital, the stress he was laboring under evidently spilled over into the hospital's parking lot one day in the form of a row the precise nature of which has not been handed down to posterity, but which may have bordered on fisticuffs. In any case it involved behavior uncharacteristic of McGovern and sufficiently reprehensible to draw down an antiseptic reprimand from the hospital:

April 5, 1953
Dear Dr. McGovern:

The altercation in which you engaged in the Hospital parking lot, was discussed briefly by the Executive Committee because of the fact that unfavorable publicity to the Hospital might have resulted. The Committee is aware that you are fully conscious that such episodes are regrettable and considers the subject closed.

John A. Washington, MD
Chairman, Executive Committee of the Medical Staff.[97]

The parking lot incident is evidently doomed to remain a mystery. It occurred long before Kathy's time, and I have not been able to uncover anyone who remembers it; there is only the bare trail in the correspondence.

But it was clearly the work of a man who had a temper and was ready to stand his ground.

Losing his father during this period and being increasingly unhappy with his situation at George Washington University probably precipitated an action more important than a parking lot altercation. The next year McGovern would pen Davison a brief update that he was on his way to Tulane University School of Medicine in New Orleans. "There is no question in my mind," he wrote on June 10, 1954, "that the Associate Professorship with Ralph Platou at Tulane, with the opportunities that exist there, represents a real improvement in my situation."[98]

Within months McGovern would learn from Davison that one of his favorite pediatrics professors at Duke, Grant Taylor, had just accepted an offer to go to Houston to head the pediatrics department at the new University of Texas M. D. Anderson Hospital and Tumor Institute (now the University of Texas M. D. Anderson Cancer Center).[99] McGovern went on about his business, but he took notice of this move and of the new medical center, which was gaining national attention.

The Big Easy (1954–1956)

Three young physicians had founded Tulane University School of Medicine in New Orleans more than a century before McGovern's arrival. The school opened in 1835 with classes taught in locations across the city, including Charity Hospital, the second oldest public hospital in the United States.[100] Only Bellevue Hospital in New York could claim to be older, having opened its doors only six weeks earlier, on March 31, 1736. The Hôpital des Pauvres de la Charité or Hospital for the Poor would in time simplify its name to Charity Hospital. Needless to say, the colorful French settlement of New Orleans, founded in 1718 by Jean-Baptiste le Moyne, Sieur de Bienville, on a crescent-shaped land mass in a bend of the Mississippi River, had plenty of poor.[101] Finding early French settlers in North America willing to move to the new Crescent City was much more difficult than originally planned. When traditional methods of flyers and advertisements failed, the French government turned to a more direct solution by snatching "recruits" for the new city from French jails and streets and loading them onto ships. Many died en route and many more fell hard to the ravages of infectious diseases such as yellow fever that afflicted the new settlement in epidemic proportions.

It took the foresight of Jean Louis, a French shipbuilder who worked in New Orleans, to leave funds in his will to establish a hospital. Events moved uncustomarily fast for New Orleans after the death of Jean Louis a year later, on January 21, 1736. The hospital charter was created that very day, and within four months the hospital at Chartres and Bienville streets, a refitted home with curtains hung to keep the mosquitoes out, was admitting patients. In less than a month the new hospital was deemed at capacity and overcrowded.[102]

Hurricanes, fires, even a duel between doctors (both missed)[103] provide a colorful history of the hospital that began in a home and moved five different times until it was rebuilt on Canal Street in 1939—the year John P. McGovern graduated from Woodrow Wilson High School and was accepted at Duke.[104] In 2005, a hurricane named Katrina delivered a knock-down blow to the city and closed the hospital. Planning for a somewhat controversial new state-owned $1.2 billion academic medical center is now underway.

The move to New Orleans, a city rich in tradition and Old South charm, must have been a culture shock for Tulane's newest associate professor of pediatrics. But he made the transition. One of his first medical students, John Fordtran, remembers McGovern as an excellent teacher in the clinics who treated his students generously and was a man of great personal appeal: "He treated me as a colleague, rather than a student, and we became close friends. We worked on experiments that Jack allowed me to publish as a sole author in the *Tulane Medical Bulletin*. Jack was a very considerate and thoughtful man . . . and he had real style. He was handsome and charming. He kept a great suntan, easily nurtured in one of the longest and blackest convertibles I ever saw. . . . In retrospect, he was in 1955–56, a lot like John F. Kennedy in the early 1960s."[105]

At the time, Charity Hospital had two separate programs, one at Tulane and the other at Louisiana State University, located eighty miles up Interstate 10 in Baton Rouge. It was on the Tulane service that McGovern started his first allergy clinic for children at Charity Hospital. To say the hospital was busy would be an understatement. James Bridges, a resident in pediatrics training with McGovern in 1954, recalls that while the hospital had a bed capacity of 3,300, it was not uncommon to find up to 4,500 patients being cared for at any one time. "There were times when we had to put two children in one bed. Twenty-bed wards became forty-bed wards. The outpatient clinics were enormous, averaging 5,000 patients per day."[106]

Actually, this was an improvement over the Great Depression years of the 1930s, only two decades before McGovern arrived as a new associate professor. In 1936 Charity's annual admission rate of 70,400 patients exceeded that of Cook County, Bellevue, and Los Angeles County hospitals—each averaging between 65,000 and 70,000 annual admissions.[107]

The hospital was perpetually overcrowded in large part because Louisiana's infamous governor, Huey Long, had proclaimed that all indigent patients in the entire state should be cared for there. Following the governor's orders, the hospital's 1935 annual report to the board shows a listed bed capacity of 1,814 and an actual daily patient bed census of 2,781.[108]

One resident physician working at Charity Hospital when McGovern arrived was John E. Salvaggio (1933–1999). Salvaggio would eventually become Tulane's vice-chancellor for research and clinical director for the clinical research program. Salvaggio's book, *New Orleans Charity Hospital: A Story of Physicians, Politics, and Poverty,* addresses the hospital's colorful history and further paints a vivid picture of the conditions McGovern would have worked under as he led his students on rounds during the mid-1950s:

> The wards were severely overcrowded and poorly staffed. On one twenty-bed medicine ward, I invariably cared for thirty-five to forty patients, most of whom were extremely ill. Patients were placed on "rollers" between the beds. . . . I remember as many as eight patients dying in a forty-bed ward in a single night. The clinics were also extremely overcrowded, just as they are today. . . . When residents were not on call during "off nights," some clinical research could be done. The hospital's reputation for practical hands-on patient care experience was good, but wards and clinics were overcrowded and under staffed, and there was seldom time for scholarly pursuits.[109]

Through it all, McGovern set a hard-driving pace that required late nights in the laboratory where he conducted research, prepared manuscripts for publication, and served as editor of hospital medical publications. By night and in spare moments he practiced his presentations for the growing number of professional organizations that had welcomed him into their membership.

While most young physicians struggled to manage the demands of clinical loads, McGovern seemed to flourish and to learn in this trial by fire to organize and manage his time more efficiently than might otherwise have been necessary. He had taken seriously Osler's advice to medical students to "live your life in day-tight compartments,"[110] and doing that had become habitual to him. Throughout his life he was able to compartmentalize and manage tasks with sharp focus and minimal distraction.

As Davison had predicted, Tulane offered many opportunities for McGovern's talent and compulsive drive. In its Department of Medicine McGovern found Vincent Derbes, who had more than a passing interest in asthma and the field of allergy. Derbes proved a mentor and a sounding board for McGovern's many interests. One of Derbes's studies addressed grain dust and allergenic air pollutants in and around New Orleans. A special asthma clinic was set up to investigate the numbers, the epidemiologic picture of suspected relationships between atmospheric pollution and outbreaks of allergies in the community.[111]

McGovern was delighted to be working with faculty invested in such studies and to be able to run his own children's clinic while teaching the next generation of Tulane physicians. By now his reputation as a triple hitter was established; he was widely recognized as highly proficient at teaching, patient care, and research. Additionally, his broad interests—in rare books, medical history, and professional organizations (in which he worked nonstop)—set him apart from most other high achievers of his day.

But he also recognized that he needed to focus his interests instead of letting them scatter in all directions and diminish the impact of his life's work. He wrote to Davison on May 25, 1955, "Dr. Derbes put me up for the American College of Allergists and the American Academy of Allergists. Have quit fooling around with bits of work in many areas now for the most part, and our research is limited to immunology with relationship to allergy."[112] Two months later his report to Davison was even more direct. "I'm an allergist now."[113] McGovern not only took the allergy boards, he passed them without the advanced training of a fellowship in the field (now typically required), a rare feat that few at the time attempted and fewer still achieved.

For McGovern this new identity as an allergist was not a departure from pediatrics. Although he now took on adult patients as well, he would continue to treat children as an allergist. Allergy was a field with direct application to his pediatric patients. But in financial terms, he diversified.

As for getting married, he would put that off another six years, but life was indeed very good for the young bachelor physician who drove a convertible, belonged to local country clubs, and enjoyed the charm of the city's French Quarter and Cajun food. Moreover, he found New Orleans to be a city where his beloved Tabasco sauce adorned the tables of even the finest restaurants.

His letters home continually update his mother on his work, and they document his continuing vigilance about her well-being. Lottie Brown McGovern sewed curtains and assisted her son from afar as he tended meticulously to the details of decorating his apartment at 2203 St. Charles Avenue. She advised him not just on the quality but on the size (to the inch) of the rug. On July 9, 1955, he reported back to her on their success:

> You should see my apartment now. All painted—the light green with gray that you picked out. The pictures are hung. I bought a new green wool rug. It was on sale at Holmes. Top quality make, but instead of 9x12 it was 9x11¼. . . . The size is just perfect in here. Everyone wishes they had gotten one like this instead of cotton. It vacuums well, etc. It is not real dark, nor yet light. . . . Have you started on the drapes? Everything else is very "spick & span" here.[114]

Today the apartment building is a popular hotel in the heart of the city's Garden District, where century-old oaks are draped in Spanish moss (and occasionally Mardi Gras beads), and the clanging bells of the St. Charles Trolley make busy urban background music.

The bird with four wings might have had six or eight wings at this point; McGovern was active on many fronts. He mastered the art of multi-tasking and took the best lessons of Osler and Davison to another level. Borrowing Osler's advice to "live neither in the past nor in the future, but let each day's work absorb your entire energies and satisfy your wildest ambition,"[115] McGovern required that every opportunity count toward multiple outcomes. An invitation to speak in Washington at a professional meeting was an opportunity to visit with his mother, attend events, network at the Cosmos Club, and compare notes with fellow physicians.

Networking was an acquired skill and McGovern had learned it from the best. His sphere grew, and his infectious enthusiasm attracted attention and interest even in the crowd of compulsive achievers in which he moved. He took center stage and always delivered. If he was asked for one idea, he delivered three.

As McGovern's life got busier with new professional organizations, papers in press, research projects planned and ongoing, and the like, his letters to Davison grew longer. Despite Davison's polite suggestions to his protégé that he would prefer shorter, more succinct letters to the single-spaced, multi-page missives he got, McGovern's letters only grew longer as his brain teemed with his growing interests, activities, ambitions, and enthusiasms.

McGovern saw even the rare vacation as an opportunity to squeeze in more work: "I am leaving August 11 for South America," he writes Davison. "How about that! Am taking my vacation as Ship doctor. Should be a great experience, much fun and a chance to catch up on some reading."[116]

The trip took McGovern to St. Thomas and beyond. As ship's doctor he received free passage and sat at the captain's table, thus replaying part of his Duke fellowship sojourn to London and Paris via the SS *America* in 1949. This trip was on the Delta Line's SS *Del Sud,* and the young ship's physician dressed in full white uniform must have cut a sharp figure.

But it was a working vacation. He wrote his mother on April 14, 1955, "The trip so far has been marvelous, and, believe it or not, I really even enjoy the work. The first 3 days out I had considerable to do, checking the final supplies and a number of cases of sea-sickness. The second day out I had a number of the crew with hangovers from their stay in port and several burns from working in the boiler room. Since then all has been relatively quiet from the professional side."[117]

In the same letter he reported that he had "made good friends with the Captain and other officers as well as the passengers. They all seem to have taken a real liking to me as I have been most conscientious in my duties." The twenty-four children on board no doubt found the ship's doctor and his magic tricks, which included his old stand-by, pulling quarters out of the air, a great treat. But McGovern was attentive to vacationing, too, and he took note of what he saw. "Passing through the Bahamas Straits was really a thrill for me. We could see Hispaniola (Haiti and the Dominican Republic) and Tortuga Island, the land of the old pirates."[118]

As he had on his travels six years earlier to Paris and London, he sat at the captain's table and once again found himself mingling with the ship's officers and wealthy passengers and dining with them on filet mignon with champignon sauce, fried soft shell crabs, roast prime rib of beef au jus, baked banana with rum sauce, and a ship's favorite—butterscotch pudding with whipped cream.[119]

Never one to waste an opportunity, the multi-tasking McGovern informed his mother that he also found time in the day for research: "Am having good success with the pollen counts, which take very little of my time."[120]

While images of mysterious lands and swashbuckling pirates captured his imagination by day, by night McGovern found ample time to catch up on his reading. Buried in the backlog of medical journals he had brought aboard was a copy of *Time* magazine dated December 13, 1954. Its cover featuring Ernest Hemingway must have seemed out of place in the stack of dog-eared learned journals he kept at his bedside. But inside that magazine was an article that caught his eye. It was about a new hospital in Houston, a cancer hospital called the "Pink Palace of Healing." The story was short but direct, and from the very first line it grabbed his attention—"The most modern, most ingeniously designed hospital in the US is the University of Texas' new M. D. Anderson Hospital and Tumor Institute in Houston."[121]

Little could he know that this one short article in a lay magazine would frame the next chapter in his life.

Tanned, handsome, charming, and dressed in his white ship's-officer uniform, the young physician had surpassed even his own expectations. He was now thirty-three years old and rising faster than those around him could entirely grasp. Yet John P. McGovern had only begun to stretch his wings.

Chapter Four

The Texas Medical Center of Houston

THE CREATION OF THE Texas Medical Center during the early 1940s is an interesting story in itself—one that frames Jack McGovern's life from the day he arrived in Houston in the spring of 1956 until he died. Long before McGovern went to Houston, men like George Hermann and Monroe Anderson had made their fortunes there, and they had given back repeatedly to the city they loved. They had provided a template for both civic pride and citizenship, and McGovern respected it deeply. Their stories were among his favorites because they gave back to the city that had provided them great opportunities. Perhaps the example of their generosity contributed in some small way to his own.

The Texas Medical Center emerged during World War II from a mosquito-infested forest that, being over three miles from Houston's downtown, was considered too far out to be of value. Today it is one of the nation's great medical treasures. It includes twenty-one academic institutions and fourteen hospitals that collectively coordinated 7.2 million patient visits in 2012. At this writing the center has more than 106,000 employees in addition to 49,000 students training in the life sciences. It is a medical city very different from the tranquil forest that the two bachelors who developed it knew in their lifetimes.[1]

Two Bachelors and a Vision

Monroe Dunaway Anderson (1873–1939) died in Houston the year Jack McGovern graduated from Woodrow Wilson High School. At the time of his death, Anderson had a personal fortune estimated at $20 million.[2] But he had not always been a rich man. In fact, he had started out a bank teller in the small Tennessee town of Jackson. Anderson was not unlike the famous young banker George Bailey, portrayed by Jimmy Stewart in the classic 1947 movie *It's a Wonderful Life*.[3] He was considered one of the most trustworthy young men in Jackson, and, sitting behind the teller's window of Peoples National Bank, he had a front-row seat on the world of finance, where he watched and learned as others made good and bad decisions that separated financial success from failure.

Monroe's older brother Frank was not much interested in sitting at a desk. Frank's big break came when the James Monroe Clayton family moved to Jackson from Tupelo, Mississippi. The Claytons had deep roots in cotton farming and commerce, and when Frank Anderson met the Claytons' son Will, the dream team of cotton merchandizing was born. Will took action on his dream when he left Jackson for New York, to gain invaluable experience there working for the American Cotton Company. In time Will Clayton and Frank and Monroe Anderson finalized their plans to start their own cotton merchandizing company with $9,000, each contributing a third.[4] On August 1, 1904, Anderson, Clayton & Co. was launched.

Each partner brought special skills to the new company. The affable Frank Anderson, at thirty-six, was the senior member of the group and emanated a no-nonsense love of the business that contributed daily to the company's good reputation among cotton farmers and ginners. Monroe, thirty-one, but seasoned beyond his years, brought his financial experience. Will Clayton, at twenty-four the youngest of the group, provided his New York American Cotton Company experience, which included both negotiation skills and essential contacts with key people in New York City and Europe. In 1905 Will's brother, Ben Clayton, only twenty-two at the time, also joined the new business and brought with him his extensive knowledge of railroads and transportation.[5] Ben had been a stenographer for the top executives in New York at the American Cotton Company and was as good at listening and learning from the best in the business as he was at transcribing their meetings and correspondence.

The company began operations in Oklahoma, where cotton was more than abundant, but the young entrepreneurs soon recognized that Houston, down on the Texas Gulf Coast, was the place to be. The hurricane of 1900 that had devastated Galveston, the main port in the state, leaving more than six thousand dead,[6] had made Houston the state's center of commerce. In 1904 Houston undertook an ambitious project, financed by federal funds, to cut a ship channel to within four miles of downtown. In the Oval Office ten years later, President Woodrow Wilson pushed a button connected by telegraph to the banks of Houston's Buffalo Bayou and fired a ceremonial cannon signaling the official opening of the Houston Ship Channel.[7]

As ships bound for destinations around the world steered into the new port, Anderson, Clayton & Co. emerged as one of the biggest and most successful cotton merchandizing firms in the world. In time the partners would centralize operations in Houston, and the company's Houston workforce would number nearly eight hundred people, most of whom Monroe knew by first name.[8]

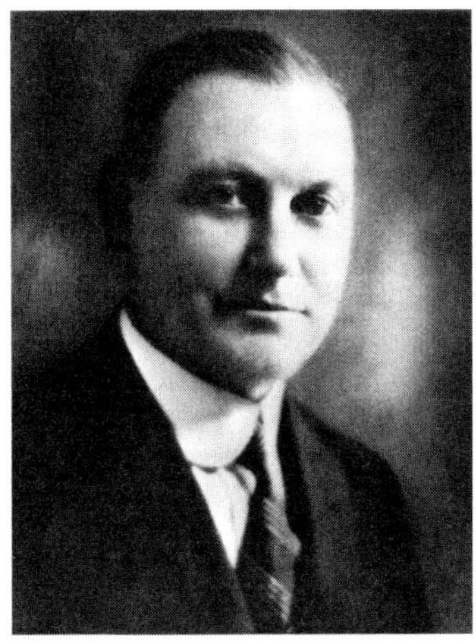

FIGURE 4.1 Monroe Dunaway Anderson (1873–1939) left his fortune to a foundation that launched a medical city from the forest behind George Hermann's hospital.

Monroe Anderson's personal savings, approaching $20 million in the 1930s—in the years of the Great Depression, no less—presented a pleasant problem for the other partners, who now included Lamar Fleming, a trusted colleague of Will Clayton's, who also had worked at the American Cotton Company. Together, the partners had an agreement that if one of them died, the others would buy out his interest at book value. But the tax laws at the time made that agreement impossible to keep without liquidating the company. One solution to the problem would be to create a foundation in Monroe's name.[9]

On June 9, 1936, the M. D. Anderson Foundation was created, and Anderson's trusted attorneys, Colonel William Bates and John Freeman of the Houston law firm Fulbright and Crooker (now Fulbright and Jaworski, LLP) turned their attention to fulfilling Anderson's directives to distribute funds for the good of the community, which included "the promotion of health, science, education, and advancement and diffusion of knowledge and understanding among people."[10]

The death of Monroe Anderson in 1939 from complications following a stroke meant that Bates and Freeman were now on their own in deciding how to fulfill Anderson's aspirations. Should they build a hospital, a clinic, or something much bigger? Houstonians were more than willing to provide their ideas, and the foundation was bombarded with a community wish list that included everything from a circus show to an amusement park.[11]

Fortunately for Houston and for health care on a global scale, both Bates and Freeman were up to the job and were as tenacious as they were faithful to Monroe's dream. So was Houston banker Horace Wilkins, who had been added as a trustee after Anderson's death. These men set their sights very high—they would build a medical city. The next step involved finding land, and a frugal Houstonian who had died more than two decades earlier provided some essential inspiration.

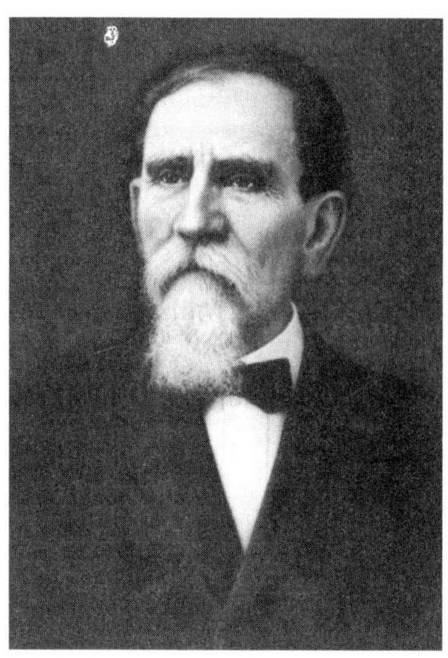

FIGURE 4.2. George Hermann (1843–1914), who willed part of his fortune to build a charity hospital for Houston.

George Hermann (1843–1914), like Monroe Anderson a lifelong bachelor, had made his Houston fortune off lumber, real estate, small cattle operations, and thirty acres of "blackjack" land he had bought for thirty-five cents an acre during a poker game. Located just north of Houston, the land was considered of little value and Hermann is said to have offered to trade it for a horse and a mule or twenty-five cents an acre. Luckily for him, he found no takers, as this was the site of the early Humble Oil Field, and the frugal bachelor with holes in his favorite sweater was soon making $50,000 a week in royalties.[12] Others would cash in as well. Upon hearing of the find, two young men a hundred miles away in Beaumont, William Stamps Farish and Robert E. Lee Blaffer, decided to form a drilling partnership, launching a company we now know as ExxonMobil.[13]

Just four months before his death from stomach on cancer October 21, 1914, at age seventy-one, Hermann gave Houston 285 acres of land for a park.[14]

The idea had come from Hermann's one vacation—an extravagant adventure for the penny-pinching millionaire who traveled to Switzerland in June of 1885 to find his long-lost Swiss relatives in Davos. Passing through New York City on his way abroad, he saw Central Park, admired its beauty, and decided that Houston should also have a park, to be named after him.[15] While Houstonians would benefit from the park he donated June 7, 1914 (after his death the 285 acres increased through additional gifts from his estate to 400 acres),[16] his search for relatives was less than successful; the ones he located had learned he was a rich Texan, and they wanted in on the money.[17] He hurried back to Houston, never to search for relatives again. After he died his Swiss relatives would pursue their claims on his fortune through a series of lawsuits, all unsuccessful; they never collected a penny of Hermann's fortune.

In years to come, Jack McGovern would give more than $6 million of his wealth to improve George Hermann's park by adding the McGovern Children's Zoo and McGovern Lake. Sharing Hermann's vision, McGovern would often say that the park and the zoo were places where families could enjoy each other's company and where children of all races were "colorblind" and could play together for the pure joy of play.[18]

Hermann wanted his city to have a charity hospital. He provided for one in his will, bequeathing the land and a large portion of his $2.6 million estate for a public hospital—"for the benefit of the poor, indigent and infirm residents of the City of Houston."[19] Hermann Hospital opened to citywide fanfare and celebration in 1925. Across the street was another monument built by another wealthy Houstonian, William Marsh Rice. He had left his money to create an institution of higher education that opened in 1912 and is known today as Rice University.[20]

In the early 1940s the Anderson Foundation trustees—Bates, Freeman, and Wilkins—saw the 134-acre forest sitting behind Hermann Hospital and across the street from the young Rice Institute very differently from those who considered it a mosquito-infested wasteland too far from downtown Houston to be of value. Their vision was Texas-sized and involved purchasing the land from the city and filling it with medical institutions. They would jumpstart this vision with a very special hospital along with a medical school. In time, other hospitals would follow.

In 1941, plans to establish a new cancer hospital and division of cancer research, to be built and operated by the University of Texas, were introduced by the Forty-Seventh Texas State Legislature, through House Bill 268.[21] Bates and Freeman moved quickly to convince Texas legislators and the University of Texas that Houston was the place for the new hospital

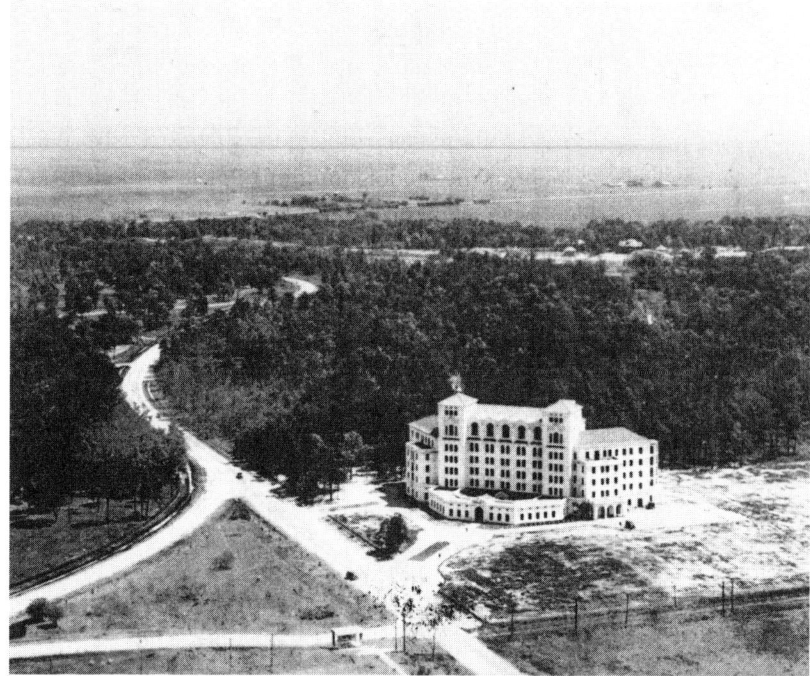

FIGURE 4.3. Hermann Hospital in 1925 and the forest Monroe Anderson's foundation would transform into one of the largest medical centers in the world.

and that the facility should be named after the foundation's namesake, Monroe Dunaway Anderson, or just M. D. Anderson for short. They would provide land and match the state's $500,000, but first they needed to secure that land from the city, and doing so required approval of a city-wide referendum by the citizens of Houston.[22] A full-page advertisement in the *Houston Post* appearing December 13, 1943, urged citizens to vote for the new medical center.[23] Voter turnout was light, but the measure passed, and at a cost of approximately $3,000 per acre, the Texas Medical Center was born.

The M. D. Anderson Foundation trustees next turned their attention to acquiring a medical school. The University of Texas Medical Branch (UTMB), sixty miles to the south on Galveston Island, had opened its doors in October 1891 as the medical department of the new University of Texas in Austin, the first medical school in Texas. UTMB had resisted moving the Galveston campus to Houston since the 1920's.[24] So Bates and Freeman headed 229 miles north to Dallas to convince Dean Walter H.

Moursund (1894–1959) and the Baylor University College of Medicine to join the new enterprise in Houston. Baylor's quarreling faculty in Dallas was at that time making plans to build a new school on land offered by the Southwest Foundation—a foundation with trustees who insisted on having an active hand in how the medical school operated. Baylor had already signed an agreement before coming to appreciate the extent of the restrictions that, Dean Moursund wrote in his history of Baylor, "made many pause to wonder if the Southwestern Medical Foundation wanted Baylor University College of Medicine in its medical center or if the foundation wanted to operate its own medical college in the center. Other medical colleges had become an integral part of other medical centers without sacrificing their university affiliation or their administrative control."[25]

Bates and Freeman stipulated no such requirements and sealed the deal in Houston with a gift of land and $1 million. Baylor's medical school dean saw his faculty undergo the equivalent of mitosis, as half of them elected to go with him to Houston to establish the Baylor University College of Medicine (changed to Baylor College of Medicine in 1969), and the other half stayed in Dallas to later become the University of Texas Southwestern Medical School (UT Southwestern).[26]

The University of Texas Board of Regents' search for someone to lead the new cancer hospital took them to a young surgeon named Randolph Lee Clark, a native of Hereford, Texas, who had earned his medical degree at the University of Virginia with graduate training at the Mayo Clinic. During the search for Clark, Ernest Bertner, a capable physician who had trained at the UT Medical Branch in Galveston, assumed interim leadership of the hospital. Bertner played a key role in the growth and organization of the medical city and served as first executive director of the medical center (the executive director's role is similar to that of mayor, with community oversight but no direct administrative control over individual institutions).

Lee Clark was just the person the University of Texas regents needed to build the new hospital. He was recruited from Jackson, Mississippi, where he had set his surgical career in motion following a distinguished military career as an air force lieutenant colonel and consultant to the surgeon general. He practiced the words of the plaque he placed front and center on his office desk—advice from his father, a teacher and school administrator who co-founded what is today Texas Christian University: "Make No Small Plans."

As a medical student, Lee Clark had once hitchhiked through Georgia with his college roommate, Jack Worsham, on their way back to Virginia from summer jobs in the wheat fields of North Texas. Sleeping peacefully (and economically) on the grounds of Emory University, the two awoke one dawn to the brilliant pink glow of a hospital building reflecting the bright morning sun. The image of that hospital gleaming in the morning light was something Clark would never forget. He was inspired; he pledged to himself then and there that if he ever could, he would build a hospital with the same stirring radiance of sunrise and hope.[27]

His chance to build his own hospital came on August 1, 1946, when he was named the new director and surgeon-in-chief of the University of Texas M. D. Anderson Hospital for Cancer Research (now the University of Texas M. D. Anderson Cancer Center). The hospital had begun in temporary quarters, the former home of former secretary of state James Baker's grandfather, Captain James A. Baker (1857–1941). With formal dedication ceremonies led by Bertner on February 17, 1944,[28] the Baker estate, also known as The Oaks, had seen its first patient several weeks later, on March 1.[29]

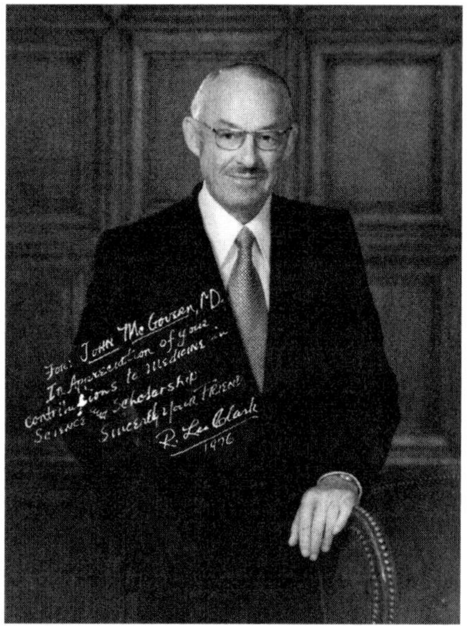

FIGURE 4.4. Randolph Lee Clark, who built M. D. Anderson.

Upon his arrival in 1946, Clark immediately bought several chickens and some poultry cloth for a pen and established the hospital's first experimental animal division out back in the estate's carriage house. In the basement of the greenhouse he established an experimental colbalt-60 unit as an early test of the emerging treatment we now know as radiotherapy.[30]

Clark, a barrel-chested all-American college wrestler in his day, was known to crawl into the home's attic to fix water pipes between surgeries. By night he could be found inspiring community groups with enthusiastic descriptions of his plans for the new cancer hospital to be built in the forest behind George Hermann's hospital and down the street from Baylor's planned medical school.

M. D. Anderson was not the only new hospital in temporary quarters. Baylor's dean Walter Moursund had found temporary quarters for his medical school in an old Sears, Roebuck building on Buffalo Drive (now Allen Parkway). Classes were first convened on July 12, 1943. High among the dean's priorities was recruiting a chairman of surgery, someone with surgical and administrative skills of the highest caliber. Moursund and his faculty found their talented surgeon in New Orleans at Tulane's Charity Hospital—a young cardiovascular surgeon of Lebanese decent named Michael DeBakey. He was known for his stellar talent and perfectionist style. Tulane's surgical residents were mesmerized by DeBakey's talent but feared the forbiddingly high expectations that earned him his nickname, Black Mike.[31] DeBakey had been a star student of Tulane's chairman of surgery, Alton Ochsner, and had risen quickly among faculty ranks. His extraordinary skills and innovations in cardiovascular surgery would make him an international legend in medicine, and a force along with such names as Bates, Freeman, Bertner, and Clark, who set the new Texas Medical Center on a world-class trajectory.

Not to be left out of the story is a brilliant dean of the city's Texas Dental College, Frederick C. Elliott (1893–1986). Elliott, born in Pittsburg, Kansas, had intended to be a pharmacist like his father, but switched his interests to dentistry and enrolled at the Kansas City Dental College, where he excelled. Elliott opened his dental practice in the city's Wirthin Building. There he became acquainted with a promising but unknown young cartoonist on the second floor, who went by the name of Walt Disney.[32]

Elliott arrived in Houston in 1932 to turn the Texas Dental College around, convert it from a proprietary school to an academic health component of the University of Texas (1943), and build a new dental school in the forest next door to Clark's cancer hospital. With that accomplished, following Bertner's death in 1950 Elliott would be named director of the Texas Medical Center and would guide its design and growth from concept to medical city.

So Clark arrived in Houston in 1946 to lead the cancer hospital and DeBakey arrived in 1947 to chair surgery and lead the Baylor College of Medicine. Then Grant Taylor came from Davison's Duke in 1955 to take charge of the newly opened cancer hospital's pediatrics service and educational programs.

Bates and Freeman's forest had been transformed by the state's new hospital, Baylor's new medical school, and Hermann Hospital on the northwest corner. If you build it they will come; and the building of what would become a medical city like no other had begun. Soon one of the largest medical libraries in the country would rise, and other medical facilities would follow.

Like Bertner, Elliott worked closely with Bates, Freeman, and Wilkins as the early trustees steered the medical center through its adolescence. In time the rapid growth and economic impact of the center demanded more community-wide involvement, and a thirty-three member community board of directors evolved—a board that would in the future include among its ranks famed Watergate prosecutor Leon Jaworski, former President George H. W. Bush, and the cream of the crop of talented Houston business and civic leaders. Today the board shares the same pride in running the expansive medical city that Bates and Freeman shared in creating it.

Ernest Bertner and Fred Elliott would be impressed that in contemporary times, under the leadership of Richard Wainerdi, who retired in December 2012 after twenty-eight years of service, the medical center has tripled in size and now includes fifty-four institutions.[33] To put that in perspective, it has been said that if you were to pull the Texas Medical Center out of Houston today, this medical metropolis would rank as the eleventh largest downtown in the United States.[34]

Six decades ago, as World War II raged across Europe, the fledgling medical center consisted of just two institutions, but Monroe Anderson's trustees had much bigger ideas. Their continued offers of land and funding sealed the deal as the thirty-three-bed Methodist Hospital, located on San Jacinto and Rosalie near downtown Houston, chose to move to the new medical center in 1951.[35] Also in the early 1950's, the Episcopal Diocese of Texas opened St. Luke's Episcopal Hospital, which focused on adult care, and pediatricians in the community, funded by Houston oilman/entrepreneur James Abercrombie,[36] realized their dream of a dedicated children's hospital, known as Texas Children's.[37] (One of its fundraising brochures was adorned with what have become the best-known cartoon characters in the world, donated by Elliott's now famous acquaintance from Kansas City days—Walt Disney.[38]) Abercrombie was guided in his giving by Leopold

Meyer, a local Foley Brothers' retail merchant and community-wide fund-raiser who always seemed to have both the ear of Abercrombie and a long list of civic ideas.[39]

On the afternoon of March 19, 1954, Clark's cancer hospital, named in Monroe Anderson's honor, formally opened its doors for patient care with the transfer of all forty-six patients from the temporary quarters of The Oaks.[40] True to his word, Clark had achieved the uplifting glow he had envisioned for his hospital—Georgia Etowah pink marble adorned its façade. *Time* magazine called it the "Pink Palace of Healing."

DeBakey and Baylor moved into their new facilities in the heart of the forest during the summer of 1947. Throughout the mid-1950s and on into the future, the forest that had been deemed too far from downtown to be worth anything was emerging as a Texas-sized Disneyland of medicine, where the best and brightest came to embark on careers in a medical metropolis—a place where patient care, research, and medical training are available on a world-class scale.

It was Clark's pink palace of healing that captured the attention and imagination of Jack McGovern, the young Tulane associate professor of pediatrics vacationing as ship's doctor aboard the SS *Del Sud* during the summer of 1955. For the ambitious McGovern, rising fast in pediatrics, allergy, and immunology, these events in Houston were impossible to ignore. To say he was intrigued by the article and by the migration to Texas of medical talent like DeBakey, Clark, and Taylor (one of his favorite former professors at Duke) would be understatement.

McGovern's success in research and at Charity Hospital's clinics at Tulane resulted in his being drawn closer into the ranks of academic administration—a direction he clearly did not want to take.[41] But it would require only a phone call from Houston on the part of his former professor at Duke, Grant Taylor, to start the next phase of McGovern's life.

Grant Taylor and the Lure of Houston

Lee Clark, a surgeon, not only planned the bricks and mortar of his new M. D. Anderson hospital down to its façade of pink marble, he also recruited pioneering faculty who shared his belief that disciplined and innovative minds were needed to expand cancer treatment beyond surgery, which was the only treatment available in the late 1940s. Treatments such as chemotherapy and radiation therapy were soon to join the cancer hospital's armament, while recruits in research would pioneer a new understanding of the biology of the disease. Insights at M. D. Anderson about the disease and its treatment would make cancer history and help guide the development of a new specialty known as oncology.

Many of the early faculty who joined Clark had just arrived in Houston on the heels of World War II military service. Together they would transform M. D. Anderson into a state-of-the-art cancer hospital that became one of the first three National Cancer Institute-designated comprehensive cancer centers in the nation, along with Memorial Sloan-Kettering Cancer Center in New York City and Roswell Park Cancer Institute in Buffalo, New York.

In 2013, M. D. Anderson Cancer Center was named for the seventh year in a row in *US News & World Report's* annual rankings as the nation's number one hospital in cancer care—a testament to Clark's vision and early recruitment savvy that included hiring Grant Taylor.[42]

Harvey Grant Taylor (1903–1995) was the son of a San Francisco pharmacist who had sold his business to become a pioneer wheat farmer in the Canadian wilderness northwest of Calgary. At the age of five, Grant was with his family in a wagon traveling across the Canadian prairie. They were looking for the homestead his father had filed for sight unseen. "On Sunday before our departure," Taylor recalled later,

> we boarded the street car that went through Golden Gate Park, beyond the Cliff House on San Francisco Bay. . . . It was here my father gave me my first lesson in shooting a gun. We departed San Francisco for Calgary early in the spring of 1909. I was almost six years old. The railway station in Calgary was a big tent. The seats were stumps of trees and logs cut to sitting height. My father left my mother and me in the station, while he rushed to the Land Office to file on our homestead. I was all eyes and ears, for those sitting on tree stumps next to my mother and me were Indians.[43]

Grant Taylor's early childhood was an education in risk-taking and surviving in a tough environment, and from it he learned skills that would last him throughout his life. In time the family would return to California, where he would enroll in high school and then earn a bachelor's degree in mechanical engineering at San Jose State College and a master's in education at Stanford. Although he had had his eye on a doctorate in psychology, he shifted his plans to medicine and found his way to Wilburt Davison's new medical school in Durham. He graduated from Duke in 1940 at the age of thirty-seven—one of the oldest graduates in his class.[44]

While World War I had influenced Taylor's early life and brought him from the Canadian wilderness back to California, World War II would shape his medical life. At Duke, he was a Davison convert and followed in the dean's footsteps as both pediatrician and Oslerian. Then he joined Davison's faculty and helped introduce a new generation of pediatricians, including Jack McGovern, to the humanistic and patient-centered Oslerian approach to medical care.

As an Army physician during World War II, Taylor received a Bronze Star and a battlefield promotion for his work under fire on Okinawa. There he had taken charge of medical needs off the battlefield, providing care that ranged from saving soldiers bitten by venomous snakes to helping the Okinawa citizens and their children with a form of encephalitis he had never seen before—Japanese B encephalitis.

Working out of tents in the jungle, Taylor cared for the local islanders with dedication and compassion. He saw that "the Okinawans feared family separation even more than death," and he came to understand that treating the disease but not the patient, or the patient but not the family, was not enough. These lessons he carried forward with him into pediatric cancer care as he applied his compassion for people, along with his training in psychology and education, to make a difference for those in his care.[45]

One group of visitors to Taylor's wartime clinic in the jungles of Okinawa was especially memorable. They were high-level guests of Taylor's commanding officers, without a stated mission, and in Taylor's words, "They stayed with us for six days and abruptly announced their departure. I rode with them down the island to headquarters, and although I made inquiry, I received no information as to who they were or what their mission was. Such was war."[46] But shortly thereafter Taylor did find out their identity: "I learned what had transpired in Hiroshima and, ultimately, that the four mysterious visitors who had recently been assigned to our unit were nuclear physicists sent to the Pacific in connection with the bombings of Hiroshima and Nagasaki."[47] And the next phase of Taylor's medical career would be related to those bombings.

Taylor returned to the States and to Duke, where he became an associate dean and pediatrics faculty member under Davison. The year was 1949, and McGovern must have been pleased to hear that Davison had invited Taylor back to Duke.

But this return would be short-lived for Taylor, who by this time was married and had two young sons. Shortly he accompanied Davison to Washington. Now an associate dean, Taylor often accompanied Davison on Duke-related business, and this particular trip was to attend a scheduled meeting of the National Academy of Science. "Everyone I met," he wrote, "was interested in talking about the National Research Council's responsibility to initiate a program designed to study the survivors of the atomic bombs exploded over Hiroshima and Nagasaki."[48] Taylor was more than interested and he was soon at the center of the discussion. He had personally seen the devastation of Hiroshima, and he cared deeply about medical research and understanding the human biological tragedy unfolding in Japan. He cared about the loss of lives and about the chronic health issues that would follow the country for decades, affecting the entire culture.

Little was known at the time about the medical effects of irradiation on the human body. Taylor was quickly identified as the kind of physician to help find the answers—Duke-trained and military-disciplined. In 1949 he was asked by Washington to return to Japan as deputy medical director of research with the Atomic Bomb Casualty Commission in Hiroshima. He worked five years there and became the director of the commission itself, with a $2.54 million budget to develop suitable facilities, oversee research and educational programs, and recruit professional staff.[49]

A pediatrician who had such a strong skill set in treating children and was pioneering an international understanding of the dire medical effects of the new nuclear age, Grant Taylor could not escape Lee Clark's Houston-based radar screen for long. Clark was building a cancer hospital that required the best faculty talent to be found, and he especially liked experienced military physicians like Grant Taylor.[50]

In pediatrics Clark wanted someone who would rewrite the textbook on childhood leukemia and other cancers common in children, someone with compassion, a firsthand knowledge of ionizing radiation's effects on the human body, and an open mind on the question whether the harmful effects of radiation could be harnessed to destroy only the cancerous cells, with minimal damage to normal cells in proximity. In short, he wanted Grant Taylor.

As chief of pediatrics and dean of the UT Postgraduate School of Medicine, which was responsible for continuing-education programs for physicians throughout Texas, Taylor would become both a leader in developing new cancer care for children and an innovator seeking new means for educating physicians throughout the Texas Medical Center and beyond.

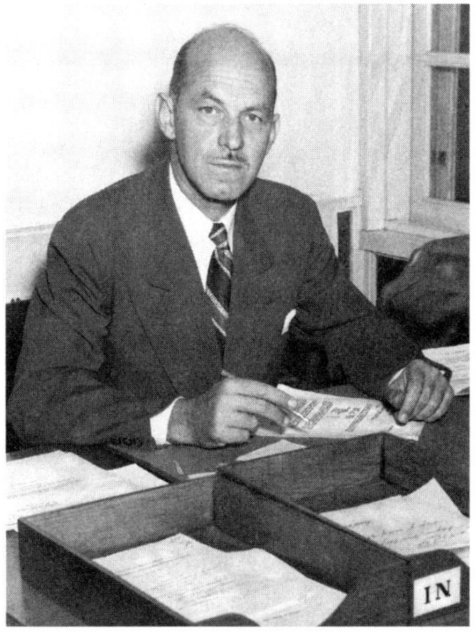

FIGURE 4.5. Grant Taylor, former head of the US Atomic Bomb Casualty Commission, went on to head the pediatrics program at M. D. Anderson.

In addition to his two positions at UT, Taylor held a clinical professorship of pediatrics at Baylor's medical school down the street. These positions constituted one of the first two joint appointments in the Medical Center's history.[51]

Perhaps it was only a matter of time before Grant Taylor picked up the phone and called Jack McGovern, his former Duke student now at Tulane. Taylor had followed McGovern closely in recent years and knew that the Texas Medical Center was exactly the kind of place where a man like McGovern could both contribute and prosper. Here he could establish a private allergy clinic near the medical city while holding academic appointments for the teaching and research that Taylor could arrange for him at institutions poised on the brink of greatness.

Houston Bound—1956

The immense opportunity that Houston offered should have made the decision to move there an easy one for a man as driven to succeed as McGovern. But it was not easy; in fact, he agonized over it, examining every pro and con exhaustively. McGovern was an ambitious man, but he was also fundamentally a careful one. He remembered all too well his first faculty appointment at George Washington University, where he had found his need for more laboratory space and support largely ignored, and where he had found administrative duties encroaching on what he meant to be his life's work (as was happening again at Tulane). He had been at Tulane only two years. It was 1956; forty was only a few years down the road. He must have felt pressure to make a commitment that would last and that he could truly build on. He did not want a false start. He did not want to make a mistake.

Nevertheless, it was clear that something special was happening in Houston—unique, once-in-a-lifetime opportunities were opening up, and he could not pass over them lightly.

Caution and opportunity were butting heads.

Osler, a role model in so many ways, had flipped a coin to determine his career move from Montreal to Philadelphia. But McGovern was leaving nothing to chance. He invested weeks in a close review of the possibilities in Houston. The process began with long conversations with Davison, Taylor, and a trusted network of pediatricians and allergists developed over the years. The rigorous decision-making at this point in McGovern's story is of more than casual interest, because it stemmed from a process that characterized the man and demonstrates the business savvy that was the engine of his future wealth, his foundation, and his immense success as founder of Houston's McGovern Allergy Clinic.

To have the faith in himself that Osler had pronounced critical to success, McGovern would break down a big decision and analyze it piece by piece, then put it back together again.[52] He did this repeatedly until all the parts of the decision made perfect sense and fit neatly together in his mind's eye. His ability to assimilate information from many sources and then to act intelligently and decisively on it would persist throughout his career and would account for much of his achievement.[53]

Although McGovern had talked to colleagues about this decision throughout the period he was making it, a meeting in Beaumont, Texas, in early 1956 seemed to turn the tide. There his inclination met with solid reinforcement from fellow allergists and, in addition, with promises of patient referrals when he got his practice going. Harold Bevil, one of the allergists McGovern sought out at that meeting, had also trained at Tulane under Ralph Platou before starting his own pediatric allergy practice in Beaumont. Bevel had a unique perspective on Tulane training and had the practical experience of having created a private allergy practice in Texas with a bird's-eye view of the medical center just ninety miles away in Houston. He confirmed Grant Taylor's original suggestion to McGovern that Houston offered unlimited possibilities.[54]

McGovern also learned of a respected allergist in Houston, Ralph Bowen, who was selling his private practice because of health issues. The Bowen Allergy Clinic was located in the family home Bowen shared with his wife on Montrose, a fashionable street just minutes from the Texas Medical Center and the faculty appointments that awaited McGovern at Baylor College of Medicine and the University of Texas Postgraduate School of Medicine.

Bowen, the assistant director of Balyeat Clinic for Allergic Diseases in Oklahoma City, had first come to Houston in 1937 to speak at the Harris County Medical Society on "Practical Management of Allergic Problems as Seen in General Practice."[55] Thereafter he moved to Houston and started his own pediatric allergy practice on Montrose Boulevard. It thrived into the mid-1950s, when Bowen's failing health forced him to sell clinic and practice shortly before his death, with the stipulation that his widow could continue to live on the property in the garage apartment behind the clinic.

The Bowen allergy clinic was a perfect practice for McGovern. Peter Kamin, a friend of Bowen's and a fellow allergist in Galveston at the time, had a special admiration for Bowen's approach to allergy care and great confidence in McGovern's ability to carry it on with continuity:

> Ralph and I spoke of a future association on several occasions and it is possible that his early death might have prevented this. He was the first to convince me that well-trained pediatric allergists could do more for allergic children than non-allergists, not only by merely caring more, giving more time and effort, but also continually learning more. This philosophy must have certainly remained in that building and was promptly evident in the life of Jack McGovern as he started his practice of allergy there.[56]

And so, after careful consideration, Jack McGovern, thirty-five years old, was Houston-bound.

Chapter Five

Building the Future

JACK WAS NO SOONER in Houston than he wrote Lottie to report on his progress and invite her down:

March 6, 1956
Dear Mother:

Please pardon the fact that this letter is typewritten, but you might have gathered from our recent telephone conversation that I am really "snowed under."

I arrived in Houston Thursday morning and now have my temporary license. I saw many interesting allergy patients Friday and Saturday and everything is just about all organized nicely. . . . I have taken over the Bowen Clinic for the practice of pediatric allergy and will teach at Baylor Medical School and the Texas Postgraduate School. Everything is very well organized so that I will no longer have to "kill myself." The girls in the Clinic here know the business very well and take a great burden off of my shoulders. I will teach twice a week over at the Medical School and will also have my laboratory so that we can continue our experiments. The two books that I had sections in are both out and I will send you reprints from the sections just as soon as I receive them.

After everything gets settled, perhaps you will be able to make a trip down to Houston. It is a very fine city. . . . I think of you many times each day. I am commuting back and forth to N.O. [New Orleans] each week until the end of the school year. Love to Aunt Sis.

Love,
Jack. A big hug and kiss!!![1]

First Clinic

Houston's Montrose Boulevard was known as "doctor's row" in the early 1950s because of the many physicians' homes located there with clinics attached. Immediately southwest of downtown Houston, the Montrose area has a history almost as old as the city itself and has been home to such notable residents as Clark Gable, Howard Hughes, Lyndon Johnson, and Walter Cronkite.[2]

It is worthy of note that Walter L. Cronkite Sr., DDS, also taught at Fred Elliott's Texas Dental College, as an assistant professor of prosthetic dentistry.[3] When they arrived in Houston, Walter Sr. helped the Elliotts find a home[4] while his son, Walter Jr., threw newspapers to their door from his bicycle as he dreamed of a career in journalism—although he probably never imagined he would one day be known as "the most trusted man in America."[5]

The history of Houston's Montrose neighborhood dates back to the early 1830s, when the Allen brothers, two real estate entrepreneurs from New York, first arrived and bought 6,642 acres of land to establish their town named for military hero and first president of the Republic of Texas, Sam Houston. They paid less than $1.50 per acre. In 1835 a widow memorably named Obedience Smith arrived in Houston from Mississippi. She brought her ten children with her to find a new life and within two years applied for a grant of land. In 1838 she was granted 3,370 acres that stretched from downtown Houston to present-day Rice University.[6]

This was prairie land. For decades its only residents were the cattle, deer, armadillos, and coyotes that roamed freely. As the city grew in the early 1900s, new neighborhoods like the Heights began to appear to the north of downtown, and Hyde Park, Cherryhurst, Courtland Place, Shadyside, Avondale, and Montrose appeared to the southwest. Streetcars, the main transportation used by 75 percent of Houstonians going to work in 1900,[7] were now reaching outward to the new suburbs. They were joined in 1908 by a growing number of Henry Ford's new Tin Lizzies or Model Ts that overnight made the newly developing suburbs across the American landscape both attractive and convenient.

The great homes of Houston clustered near Main Street adjacent to the downtown center of commerce, but Wiley Link, a former mayor of Orange, Texas, had plans to rival them. He took the name Montrose Place right out of the pages of Sir Walter Scott[8] and laid out a subdivision with four broad boulevards planted with seven train-car loads of palm trees to add a California touch. On Montrose Boulevard, Link built his own home (now the administration building of the University of St. Thomas). By the 1920s bungalows lined the streets of Montrose. They were followed by shopping centers in the 1930s and the community's own Art Deco movie theater, the Tower Theatre, built in 1936.

The Bowen Allergy Clinic became the McGovern Allergy Clinic in April 1956. The energetic McGovern wasted no time in building upon the good name and reputation of Ralph Bowen. True to McGovern's word, Mrs. Bowen, now a widow, would continue to live on the property, watched over by McGovern and his clinic staff.

The Bowen staff oriented McGovern to the patients, and in short order the McGovern Allergy Clinic was adding referrals and new patients, who were impressed by the knowledgeable and energetic young doctor and

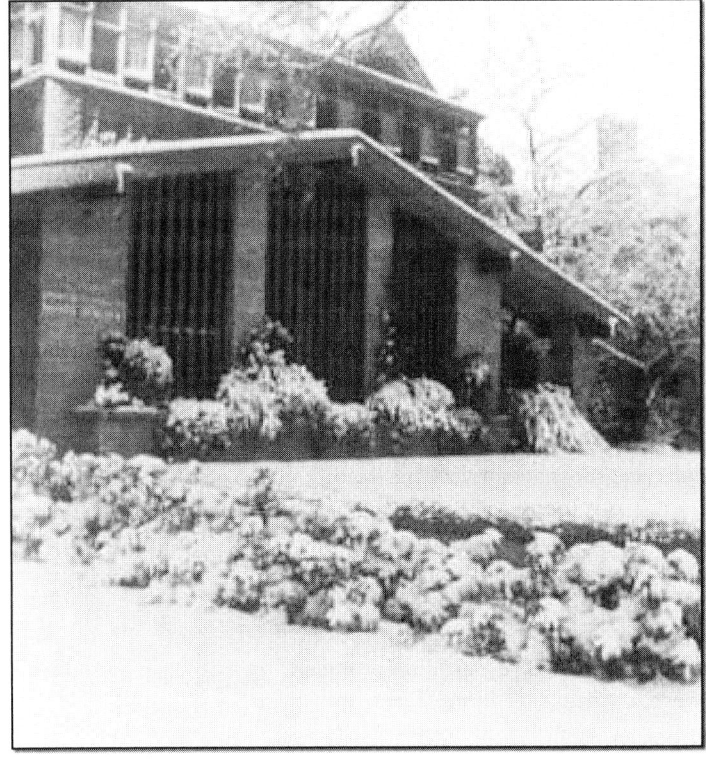

FIGURE 5.1. The first McGovern Allergy Clinic, on Valentine's Day 1961, the day of a rare Houston snowstorm.

also, no doubt, by his academic credentials in the nearby medical center, just a stone's throw down Montrose Boulevard to Main Street, Rice University, and George Hermann's park and hospital. And, in addition to making himself known among patients, McGovern found time to visit physicians' offices throughout Houston to introduce himself. Many of the new contacts he made, impressed by his confidence and no doubt pleasantly flattered by the personal visit, referred patients to him for years to come.

As McGovern had hoped, the Bowen patients stayed with the new McGovern clinic and new patients arrived daily. In the 1950s Houston, fueled by oil money, was on a rapid trajectory to become America's fourth largest city; in a few short decades it trailed only New York City, Los Angeles, and Chicago in population.[9] As McGovern foresaw, here there was no shortage of opportunity and certainly no shortage of pollen. He was soon interviewing additional staff and physicians to join his new venture. Early employees recall their first job interviews, which lasted two hours or longer and were followed by a second and sometimes third meeting. Many employees who went through those interviews remember them as epic in depth as well as length, and report that they learned as much about Dean Davison, Duke University, Osler, and the patients (who in no uncertain terms would be the focus of every part of the work at hand) as McGovern learned about them. And the interviews took the first step toward creating a close-knit family of physicians and staff who would build the McGovern Allergy Clinic into a patient care and research institution with international renown.

The narrow stairwells and creaking stairs of the old house and its cramped quarters—an upstairs bathroom had been converted into a clinic laboratory—were of little concern amid the excitement of a growing enterprise. McGovern's energy was vast and his attention to the patients was personal, as this recollection of Ada Holland, one of the early staff supporting the newly arrived McGovern, testifies:

> One of the unique privileges that we of the staff had during the early years of the McGovern Allergy Clinic was being part of the close day-to-day working relationship of Dr. McGovern with the patients. For many years Dr. McGovern undertook to and did see every new patient who came through the clinic, besides his own schedule of regular appointments. It was lively to say the least. The seemingly endless amount of

> energy that was pouring out of this capable physician during the days, months, and years was projected into the healing of patients, teaching at various schools, teaching the clinic doctors, the staff, organizing research programs, attending medical functions, setting up seminars, promoting health care, and helping any individual who needed help in any way.[10]

Maxine Mayo, one of McGovern's first secretaries, provides a verbal snapshot of the early clinic: these were "whirlwind days; dashing up and down the wooden stairway (he could always hear me coming well in advance); listening for the bang of the side door, announcing Doctor McGovern's daily arrival; the incredibly vital feeling of the Clinic with his presence; volumes of correspondence, fascinating papers, handbooks, exhibits; meeting with him at the end of each day to pore over the letters and drafts."[11]

While McGovern had left Tulane behind, he had not left his memories of exceptionally bright students who had followed him on rounds through the pediatric wards of Charity Hospital. One of those had been Theodore J. Haywood. Haywood, like many young interns and resident physicians of the day, had gravitated toward McGovern, who, "with his wealth of knowledge . . . made the difficult problems seem easy to solve. He stimulated my early interest in allergy as I worked closely with him on the wards and clinics."[12]

Haywood was in St. Simon's Island, Georgia "testing [his] wings" in pediatrics as McGovern's new clinic was taking shape in the late 1950s.[13] Interested in acquiring additional training in allergy, he placed a call to his former professor to ask for advice. McGovern flew to St. Simon's Island and told Haywood to "shake out the sand" from his shoes and go to Houston. Haywood would work side by side with McGovern during the next three decades and eventually, along with other senior associates, buy the clinic when McGovern formally retired on January 1, 1986.

Orville C. Thomas (1915–2007) first met McGovern in the summer of 1961. A pediatrician in Shreveport, Louisiana, Thomas also sought additional training in allergy. He came to Houston where McGovern was teaching postgraduate courses in allergy and immunology through his Baylor faculty appointment in the Texas Medical Center. This training prepared him to earn board certification in the field. Thomas had planned to return to Shreveport as an allergist, but McGovern had other ideas and asked him aboard as an associate at his clinic. "My acceptance of his offer," Thomas wrote, "was quick and enthusiastic." It was a decision that neither he nor his family ever regretted.[14]

Perhaps the best hire of all was a talented office manager who joined the McGovern Allergy Clinic on Montrose in its early years and proved to be an outstanding office manager who would also become McGovern's wife.

Married Man

Looking back during his twilight years, a jovial McGovern had a favorite line when asked to name the highlights of his life. He would tick them off the fingers of his left hand: (1) his friendship with Wilburt Davison, (2) the influence of Osler, (3) the day he quit smoking in 1963, (4) the day he quit drinking in 1984, and (5) the day he married a slender brunette with a head-turning smile—Kathrine Dunbar Galbreath. And then, with a practiced pause and mischief in his eye, he would add, "And not necessarily in that order."[15] The message was clear. Kathy McGovern was and would always be number one. She was, in the words of the poet, the fixed foot of his compass.

The future Mrs. McGovern's father, Joseph Galbreath, had been a Houston-area builder and architect known for his beautiful etchings and drawings. He had an artistic talent that the younger of his two daughters would remember with particular pride, given his lack of formal training in design. A Houstonian by birth, Kathy and her sister, Val, had been brought up in their parents' home on Westgate Drive, not far from the growing community of Montrose.

The Great Depression had been hard for the Galbreaths. Kathy's father had struggled to support his family, and it was always a good day, she remembers, when he found a small remodeling job of any description. For him as for others throughout the country, good days of employment were often few and far between. Joseph Galbreath died three days before Thanksgiving in 1947, at the age fifty-four. His wife took charge, went to work, and brought up her daughters, instilling in them a strong work ethic and an interest in finding careers in areas of service to the community. Kathrine would make her career in Houston's booming health sector; Val would become an elementary school teacher much beloved by her community. She is now retired in the small Central Texas town of LaGrange.

When Jack McGovern arrived in Houston in 1956, Kathy Galbreath was working as an office manager in the offices (there were two) of Dr. Goldie

Ham, a successful Houston obstetrician/gynecologist. Ham was planning to retire in 1958. Kathy remembers her as a wonderful physician, one of the few women obstetricians the city had at the time.

"When she retired," Kathy said,

> a mutual doctor friend told me that a physician over on Montrose was looking for someone. We made contact—I can't remember whether he called me or I called him. I was a trained secretary and office manager, so I did mostly front office work, which I enjoyed more, taking dictation and typing. I got the job after a very long interview and joined a fairly small staff that existed at the time including his secretary (a position I originally thought I was interviewing for), a bookkeeper who came from downstairs, two or three nurses, and Mary upstairs in the Antigen Department where he was mixing his own antigens at the time.[16]

As for the qualities she found in her new employer: he was "very focused, very intense. I took a little while to get used to that. . . . He was very intriguing, and I learned to respect him greatly. He took a little while to get used to, for me." Indeed he did; but on December 18, 1961, McGovern was making an announcement to Davison:

> I just finished calling you in Durham to tell you of an event to occur on December 20; namely, I'm going to get married. I'll bet you never thought I'd make the grade! The secretary told me that you would be out of the country until March, but I wanted you to be the first to know (my mother doesn't even know yet). The girl that I am to marry is 28 years old and has worked with me in our office for three years. She is a fine person in every way, and I know that you will like her. Am certainly looking forward to the day when I can have the great honor of introducing her to you.[17]

Dean Davison, in the midst of retiring and making the transition from dean of the medical school to a trustee of the Duke endowment, sent the bride's mother a note, somewhat belated because of his travel schedule: "I was very happy to receive the announcement of your daughter's wedding to Dr. John Phillip McGovern," he wrote. "He is one of my favorite students and I know that your daughter and he will be very happy. Please convey to the bride and groom my best wishes for every happiness."[18]

Six years earlier, in 1955, as McGovern's career was taking off at Tulane, he had itemized his recent accomplishments in a letter to Davison and had ended with, "The first thing you know, I'll be so well adjusted that I'll up and get married."[19] During his tenure on the Tulane faculty that same year, he had even contemplated marriage to his girlfriend at the time, but had broken it off, penning in explanation to his mother, "Our basic differences . . . would have seriously hurt our chances for a happy married life."[20]

It took the right person at the right time for the forty-year-old McGovern to marry. In Kathrine Galbreath he found her, and two great events in his life happened within three months of each other in 1961.

On September 15 McGovern took $10,000 from his savings and started a foundation, originally known as the Texas Allergy Research Foundation (TARF; on December 5, 1979, renamed the John P. McGovern Foundation), which would grow into a fortune.[21] Everything McGovern had touched was turning to gold; it was time, then, to invest extra income, the maximum allowed by law, and start the foundation that would enable him to give back to his community for years to come. His philosophy of giving was straightforward—"What one earns, he spends; what he wins, he loses; and what he gives, he keeps forever."[22]

And then, on December 20, he married Kathy Galbreath. His courtship had been so quiet that the marriage came as a great surprise to many of his colleagues. Ted Haywood remembers the morning when McGovern walked into the clinic and casually remarked, "I'm going to get married. Can you guess who?" Haywood adds, "And I couldn't guess."[23]

"We decided to keep it very simple," Kathy remembers, "with just the two of us at Palmer Church near the Medical Center." But in spite of the arrangements they had made, McGovern, in what can be interpreted only as successive fits of enthusiasm, "ended up asking three people to be his best man—Don Mitchell and Walt Van Sickle, two of his good friends, and his associate, Ted Haywood. They all showed up." What could have been an awkward situation was instead resolved cheerfully by the toss of a coin, which Ted Haywood won. Kathy, in the meantime, had stuck to their agreement. "I asked no one, not even my family, thinking it was just Jack and me." But any slight imperfections in the somewhat eccentric festivities were dissolved in champagne, of which some agreeable person had brought a bottle, and "we toasted in the parking lot."[24]

A week later the newlyweds left on a road trip to Florida for their honeymoon, to follow their mutual love of the ocean, sea breezes, and fishing, an outdoor sport they would share throughout their married life. Kathy remembers that "we wanted to go bone fishing, so we went down there to Islamorada and went out and went bone fishing. And then did all sorts of other fishing. We just roamed Florida. When we went down there, we cut across to the east coast and went down and came back up the west coast and drove back. We sort of fished everywhere."[25]

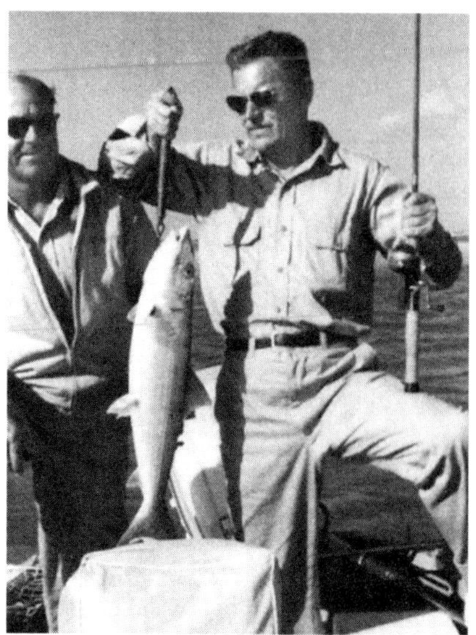

FIGURE 5.2. McGovern displaying a bonefish caught in Florida on his honeymoon in 1961. Photo by Kathy McGovern.

Over time the two would become accomplished anglers, buying a bay house on West Galveston Island, an area they especially loved. Kathy recalls that a friend, Dick Davies, had a cottage at Jamaica Beach and encouraged them to use it:

> We did take him up on the offer and we discovered West Galveston Island, which we didn't know was there. . . . We rode around while we were on vacation and found a small, one-bedroom house in Jamaica Beach on a canal and we bought it. We found that we adored it, and within the year we started looking, and that's when we found a bay-front lot with a house in Sea Isle. That's where we moved. We had the house and a lot next to it. We built a deck and a boat ramp and we put fishing lights in and we were there for about fifteen years. . . . We got to a point where I would go down every evening and fish, and if the fish got big enough, I'd go in the garage and take the crab net and hit the top of the garage to alert him as he worked in the room above. That meant they were big enough if you wanted to come down. Sometimes he would and sometimes not, but once he got down there he wouldn't stop. He loved it so much. But getting him to put down his work and come down to fish was a challenge.[26]

For McGovern, putting down work to relax had always been hard—or impossible, as his parents learned on the Thanksgiving they spent with Ziggy—but with marriage McGovern found a new if sporadic contentment. He confided as much in a letter to Davison after four years: "I was 40 years old when I finally had the good sense to marry Kathy. Since then it seems as though I have gained at least a little aequanimitas."[27] The collection of honors adorning the walls of his office and his study at home was slowly giving up space to framed photos of McGovern and Kathy flashing grins and holding up their catch—sailfish, bone fish, speckled trout, redfish, and flounder caught in Mexico, Florida, and South Padre Island. But McGovern was still McGovern, and although marriage would bring the companionship that was responsible for his increased interest in life outside of medicine, it did not undermine his professional zeal. For him, as for Osler, work was the "master word."[28] It had been too fundamentally satisfying to be surrendered. In fact, by the time he married, recognition for his work had come to him even from the White House. In 1960, Texas Senator Lyndon Johnson, who would soon become vice president to John F. Kennedy, had been given McGovern's name as a rising star among pediatric allergists and had requested his presence as a delegate to the 1960 White House Conference on Children and Youth held March 27 to April 2.[29]

McGovern found service at the national level addictive. He invested his time, energy, and eventually his wealth in many areas of interest to him, including health education in the nation's schools (through the American School Health Association) and alcohol and drug abuse prevention (through the National Advisory Council on Alcohol Abuse and Alcoholism). He also continued to support his beloved American College of Allergists. And he took on added responsibilities as a member of the board of regents for the National Library of Medicine. For each of these organizations he would hold highest office and receive highest honors for service, including the Surgeon General's Medal awarded by the most recognized physician in America of the day—C. Everett Koop.[30]

And so it is not surprising to find him writing Davison on June 7, 1965,

> This seems to have been the most demanding spring that I have ever had, what with putting on the Postgraduate Course for the American Academy of Pediatrics in March; followed by the annual meeting of the American College of Allergists in which I moderated a Round Table, gave

> two papers, served on three Committees and the Council on Research and Education, was elected First Vice President "from the floor," and was elected Associate Editor of the Annals of Allergy, to become Editor in Chief in three years; then was Chairman of the Council on Annual Sessions and Curbstone Consultations for the annual meeting of the Texas Medical Association; and made the preparations for our move on May 1st into our Clinic.[31]

To the extent that aequanimitas means taking things as they come and cultivating calm, McGovern was doomed to struggle to achieve it. He did not submit to things as they came; he shaped them. He liked action and activity and working toward goals. "I remember one greatly anticipated vacation shortly after we got married," Kathy says, "a fishing trip by car to South Texas that he reluctantly delayed week after week due to his many projects and business dealings. Finally I put my foot down and insisted we get in the car and take the vacation. I thought I had won a small victory, only to find him loading two briefcases in the car and stopping at nearly every pay phone between Houston and Brownsville as we inched our way south. I never tried that again."[32]

Although the calm that eluded her husband came naturally to Kathy, she took his inexhaustible energy and continuous activity in stride and quietly and efficiently helped him write the future stories of his life. One substantial contribution she made was in overseeing the increasing number of support staff required by the clinic. In the mid-1960s it was quickly running out of space for the ever-increasing number of patients who sought the care of the surgeon's son from Washington, DC.

Growing Pains

McGovern was not alone in the business of starting a large and successful privately owned clinic in the shadow of the fledgling Texas Medical Center. Another talented young physician, an internist, had arrived in Houston in 1949. His multispecialty clinic would become a household name in the medical center and throughout Houston.

Mavis P. Kelsey (1912–2013), a native Texan from the small community of Deport, northeast of Dallas, had earned his medical degree from the University of Texas Medical Branch in general medicine in 1936. By

September of 1939 he was married and arriving at the Mayo Clinic in Rochester, Minnesota. This was the same month and year that McGovern had arrived at Duke to commence his college studies. Kelsey's fellowship in internal medicine was interrupted on August 15, 1941, by a call to active duty as a medical officer in the US Air Force (then the Army Air Corps). His military career included promotion to flight surgeon of the Eleventh Fighter Command with assignments throughout Alaska's Aleutian Islands, including Dutch Harbor, the only American soil other than Pearl Harbor bombed by the Japanese (June 3–4, 1942).

After the war Kelsey returned to Mayo on the first day of 1946 to complete his fellowship in gastroenterology and endocrinology. While his fellowship had paid $75 a month, one year to the day later, at age thirty-four, he was offered a permanent position as a staff physician with a salary of $1,000 a month—what was then a mark of great accomplishment and prestige that young physicians at Mayo aspired to achieve and few were known to surrender.[33]

However, with his strong Texas roots and a wife from Beaumont, Texas, word of the new Texas Medical Center would pull Kelsey like a magnet back to Houston. The many prominent Houstonians who went to the prestigious Mayo Clinic for their care had taken with them word of the excitement and buzz the new medical center in Houston was generating, and Kelsey paid attention.

In addition to Horace Wilkins, the M. D. Anderson Foundation trustee who had replaced Monroe Anderson upon his death in 1939, Dr. Ernest Bertner, the interim director of the new cancer hospital and founding director of the medical city, was at the time himself a patient at the Mayo Clinic. He personally invited Kelsey to take a look at the new center being built in Houston. Lee Clark, who had also trained at Mayo, made offers to Kelsey to go to Houston and join his new cancer hospital as chief of medicine.[34] In his own book, *Twentieth-Century Doctor: House Calls to Space Medicine,* Mavis Kelsey said, "The most spectacular of my patients were Wesley and Neva West of Houston. They came in their private DC-3, the finest private plane then available. . . . He wanted me to come to Houston and practice medicine. He even offered to build me a clinic on a tract of land near the new medical center."[35]

Kelsey took his family to Houston in 1949, along with Mayo surgeon and friend Bill Seybold. Bill Leary, a brilliant Mayo internist who had passed his specialty boards in unheard-of fashion while on duty during World War II and before completing residency training, also went.[36] In 1953, Kelsey's younger brother John, a Mayo-trained gastroenterologist, joined the practice.[37] The multispecialty Kelsey-Seybold Clinic they built near the Texas Medical Center would become a success story unrivaled by any other privately owned clinic in Houston until McGovern arrived in 1956 to start his allergy practice. Kelsey's clinic, with its own radioisotope laboratory, assisted the early cancer hospital by treating all the inoperable thyroid cancers. Mavis Kelsey's private practice prospered and required larger and larger buildings near the Medical Center to house it.

As McGovern was growing his clinic on Montrose in the early 1960s, Kelsey was opening his second clinic on the corner of Southgate and Travis, right across the street from the Texas Medical Center. The land was owned by the Hannah family, who were willing to build the clinic and lease it to the growing Kelsey enterprise. Kelsey and his group were given complete control in the design and brought in the architectural firm of Wilson, Morris and Crane, known for their contemporary designs.[38]

Little could McGovern know that in ten years Kelsey would outgrow the clinic building he had opened in December 1954 (then known as the Kelsey-Leary Clinic) and that it would become available for lease. Kelsey would move farther up the street, across from Hermann Hospital, while from 1965 until 1973 McGovern would occupy the clinic building Kelsey left behind. The additional space within walking distance of the rapidly growing medical center did nothing to dim McGovern's recognition as a rising star.

But the prominent allergy clinic that had once met Kelsey's space needs now seemed small to McGovern, too, as patients increased in numbers that soon overtook the available parking, and lease agreements were about to expire. Additional land leased across the street helped for a while and added additional space for Kathy and the growing administrative staff, but only for the moment.

A bigger plan was needed. On March 7, 1971, McGovern outlined one to the now retired Davison:

> As I had mentioned to you, we must build a new clinic in that the owners of our present building had told us that our lease could not be extended beyond April of 1972. This would have left us approximately only one year, which around these parts can be insufficient time. Before leaving on

our vacation, we were able to arrange an extension until June 1972, which even so meant that we had to get off the dime and start working with the architects. Although we had already purchased the land years ago, we procrastinated and then, because of the recent poor long-term money market, purposely delayed getting into building of the clinic as long as possible. Although costs now will be greater, we will be able to make better interim interest and permanent financing loans. Actually, we would have had to do something anyway in that our parking problem is becoming ever more acute and we have ample land at the new site for any growth that might take place.[39]

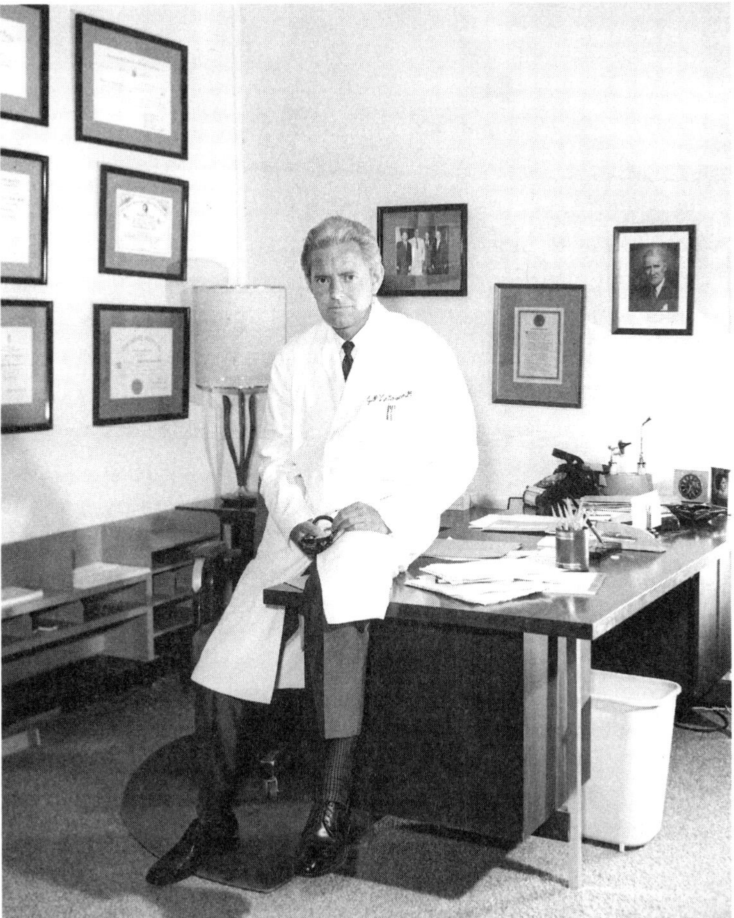

FIGURE 5.3. McGovern in his Travis Street clinic in the mid 1960s.

As McGovern's new building took shape, the early dawn would often find him standing at the construction site taking in the view. And Lee Clark could often be found standing beside him. Clark, who less than two miles away had built one of the great cancer hospitals of all time, was interested in the thinking that had gone into the design of McGovern's clinic. He was all ears about the business side of a man's constructing his own building on land he had bought years earlier.[40]

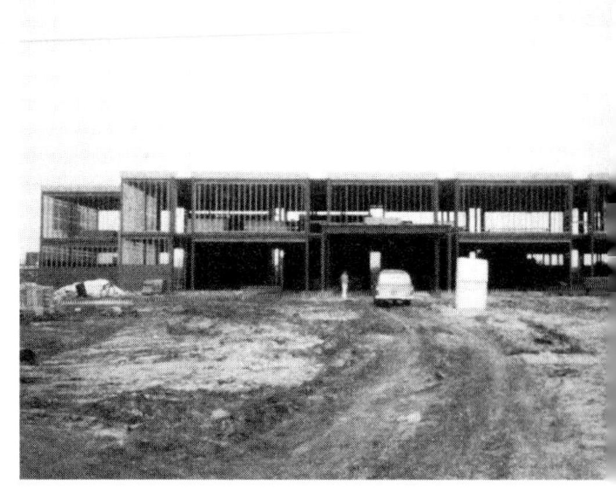

FIGURE 5.4. McGovern's new clinic under constru tion near the Texas Medical Center in the early 197c

Clark had built M. D. Anderson Hospital, the pink palace of healing, with equal attention to design, flow of patients, integration of research facilities, and continuous education of health professionals. McGovern would build his clinic with that same attention to detail. It would be a building that was patient-friendly and large enough to house both research and fellows in training, who, in increasing numbers from all parts of the country, sought out McGovern and his facilities.

The design for his new clinic included a prominent gallery and library honoring Wilburt Davison, Sir William Osler, and the history of medicine. Also prominent was a "Fellows Room" honoring the many physicians who had completed their advanced training in allergy/immunology under McGovern's watchful eye. The design was not all McGovern. True to his inclusive attitude toward staff, he asked Ada Holland, his secretary, and also Kathy, as office manager, to meet with each department in the clinic about its needs, wishes, and design suggestions. All were given access to the architects, making the new clinic building a source of pride for not only the Chief, but also his entire family of employees. In a letter announcing the near completion of the building, McGovern did not omit to update his former students, many of whom now led their own clinics and chaired departments in medical institutions around the world.

"Each day," he wrote in a letter dated June 4, 1973,

> while walking down the hall I see your fine photographs which bring back pleasant memories and the knowledge of how fortunate I have been to work with such a splendid group of colleagues and friends over the years. . . . The new Clinic is progressing beautifully. As most of you know, it will be two stories with a total of 30,000 square feet. It will contain, in addition to the waiting room, examining rooms, testing areas, clinical and antigen laboratories, etc., two complete research laboratories on the second floor across from a large library. We expect to move in September (six months late) and needless to say, hope that each one of you will come visit with us before long.[41]

In a medical city with enough ambitious and talented physicians to fill a football stadium, McGovern was an outlier who in less than a decade was a recognized name in national medical and business circles. Lee Clark, who had built M. D. Anderson from the ground up, could only be impressed as he listened in the early morning hours to McGovern's detailed explanation of the planning behind his research laboratories, patient exam rooms, Davison/Osler gallery, and second-floor office where McGovern would conduct his medical and business affairs and watch his clinic and his foundation grow beyond all expectations.

Clark, the mastermind of one of the world's great cancer hospitals, who lived by his father's advice, "Make no small plans," had certainly found a kindred spirit in Jack McGovern.

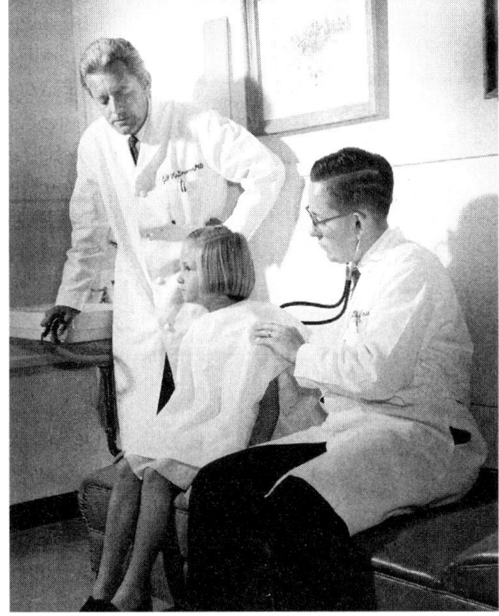

FIGURE 5.5. McGovern trained a generation of pediatric allergists. Shown here with fellow Charles Haunschild and patient, circa 1966.

Academic Pioneer

While McGovern's allergy clinic continued to prosper, the two faculty appointments he held at Baylor College of Medicine and the University of Texas Postgraduate School of Medicine should not be overlooked. Both dated back to his arrival in Houston in 1956 and both helped shape his success.

BAYLOR COLLEGE OF MEDICINE AND TEXAS CHILDREN'S HOSPITAL

On July 1, 1960, Baylor's dean, Stanley W. Olson, sent McGovern a memo stating that "the Board of Trustees has officially approved my recommendation and that of your department chairman for your appointment as Clinical Associate Professor of Pediatrics and Microbiology for the year beginning July 1, 1960, at an annual stipend of $3,600." At the bottom of the memorandum, McGovern scribbled a hurried note, a reminder to himself—"This is the third year of this Baylor appointment."[42]

Dean Olson had good reason to renew this clinical faculty appointment at Baylor. McGovern, in addition to building his own private allergy clinic, had simultaneously developed Baylor's first allergy and immunology residency and fellowship program, providing novel advanced training in a field growing rapidly in its understanding of the relationship between the allergic diseases and immunology. This program would be the first of its kind in the Texas Medical Center and a model for the advanced specialty training that others would develop for new medical specialties in years to come.

McGovern's timing was spot-on. The fields of allergy and immunology converged in the late 1960s into a specialty that would take the medical profession by storm—and would create a major shift in credibility from the turn of the century, when the term "allergy" had been shadowed by controversy. Coined in 1906 by Austrian pediatrician Clemens von Pirquet (1874–1929), the word was first used to describe the strange, non-disease-related symptoms that some diphtheria patients developed when treated with a horse serum antitoxin. (Pirquet, it should be noted, is also the father of the modern tuberculosis test named after him.[43]) The word comes from the Greek "allos" and denotes a change in original state. An allergic reaction is an altered or exaggerated reaction and the allergy patient is said to live in an altered state of hypersensitivity. Thus, an allergic reaction is the result of the body's change when it adversely responds to a harmless substance (pollen and mold are common culprits) or is induced by immune mechanisms such as too much of the allergy-provoking antibody IgE.

Focusing on the temporal characteristics of the clinical phenomena, Pirquet and his Hungarian co-worker, Bela Schick (1877–1967), demonstrated that serum sickness presented a familiar set of pathological features. They concluded that the clinical features of serum sickness were not the direct product of the antiserum but the outcome of a hypersensitive reaction characterized by "a collision of antigen and antibody."

Pirquet became the first professor of pediatrics at Johns Hopkins University, a position he held only one year (1909–1910). The position he left behind became the catalyst for Hopkins to start a pediatrics department, and it paved the way for John Howland to arrive in 1912. Tragically, Pirquet and his wife would become addicted to morphine and would take their own lives in 1929, a dark day in the history of allergy that even McGovern was surprised to learn about in 1968, nearly twenty-five years into his medical career.[44]

Pirquet's formulation of allergy helped to sustain both conceptual and practical links between immunology and medicine. In other words, immunology moved from the remote research lab to the clinic. But it took yet another sixty years to get the American Medical Association's blessing on the field as a recognized specialty.

As recently as the 1950s, a mere blink of time in the history of medicine, the clinical allergist had yet to gain the full respect of the medical profession. Not until 1966 did the American Medical Association even have an Allergy Section. Getting one was a major step toward the creation of a board and independent specialty recognition. Philip Gottlieb, a founding father and former president of the American College of Allergy and Immunology, recalls the slow rise of recognition for allergists from being considered "technicians" or "wheeze, sneeze, and itch doctors"[45] in the 1940s and 50s to becoming members of a widely recognized specialty in the early 1970s. In a videotaped presentation celebrating the American College of Allergy and Immunology's fiftieth anniversary, Gottlieb joined McGovern and other former presidents in reflecting on the organization's growth. Gottlieb had been co-chairman of the Allergy Meeting of the AMA when allergy was considered part of a miscellany. "It gave me the shivers," he said in the video, "every time I had to walk through that door with the sign in front, 'Section of Miscellaneous Topics.'"[46]

As the Vietnam war raged through the late 1960s and dominated the nation's collective attention, the headlines of medical research journals chronicled a virtual information explosion in basic research that put clinical allergists on the medical map as respected colleagues and specialists. In 1967, a husband-and-wife team of Japanese researchers, Kimishige and Teruko Ishizaka, made a breakthrough in allergy studies when they discovered the role of IgE (immunoglobulin E) protein as a key element for provoking immediate-type hypersensitivity in mammals. This was a finding that revolutionized our understanding of allergic reactions.[47] IgE is naturally produced by the body, but in greatly increased quantities by those who are susceptible to allergies. It is responsible for the majority of allergy symptoms such as anaphylaxis, hay fever, pollen asthma, and some types of eczema, insect allergy, and drug allergies. The discovery of and subsequent research into IgE helped the field of allergy study evolve from a guessing game into the well-understood and accepted immunologic science that it is today.

Also in 1967 McGovern published his first book on allergy, *Allergy and Human Emotions.* He and his co-author, former Tulane colleague James A. Knight, emphasized that no one factor is the cause of disease, and that the whole patient with all of his problems must be considered in the diagnosis and treatment of allergies.[48]

McGovern, who had once told his father that a million dollars would not get him to join the ranks of psychiatry, had, as previously acknowledged, amended his thinking over the years about the value of behavioral medicine. Now he and Knight (a psychiatrist and ordained Methodist minister) had produced a unique and head-turning book written for a broad audience of physicians. It served as a primer of the emotional dimension of allergic illnesses. McGovern's meticulous documentation distinguished the book as a scholarly work of the first order.[49]

When the American Board of Allergy and Immunology was established in 1971, it included representatives from pediatrics and internal medicine.[50] McGovern was in all the right places to lead in the new field. In March 1968 he had been elected president of the American College of Allergy and Immunology and therefore had had a direct hand in the ongoing process of obtaining board certification and recognition of specialty status. Additionally, he was well known and respected as co-editor of leading professional journals in the field and networked with leading allergists throughout the country as well as internationally. He was ready to lead.[51]

At Baylor McGovern developed and championed pioneering postgraduate training programs for physicians interested in joining the new specialty. If you were a physician wanting advanced training in allergy and immunology at this pivotal time in the specialty's advancement, McGovern's fellowship program at Baylor was the place to go. Here you could train with McGovern himself. The young allergists who followed McGovern to Baylor found unparalleled educational possibilities in his clinics. Few aspiring allergists at the time could comfortably ignore the opportunity to train with him. James Murray, one of their number, said this:

> I came into the fellowship of allergy with a firm desire to learn all I could about its science, its clinical practice, and especially the relationship between atopy and the new discoveries in the field of immunology. If nothing else, I was eager. And yet, no matter how often I arrived in the early hours of the clinic to study, nor no matter how late I'd stay, Doctor McGovern arrived first and left last. I still carry his example of hard work and diligence with me.
>
> . . . Dr. McGovern's role was one of encouraging me to study the new science of immunology while also proceeding to show me the vast diagnostic and therapeutic challenges in clinical allergy. He perceived his task as one to illustrate not only what was known, but also what was not known. . . . On many occasions there was vigorous, heated debate. . . . The Chief brought the fellows to the realization that they must know the theory, but most importantly, they must be prepared in a few short years to face allergic patients whose illnesses could range from a mild irritation to a potentially fatal disease. . . . The Chief taught me to seek to be a brilliant listener, to care about the patient, and to strive to provide the best therapy currently available.[52]

In this way, McGovern impressed upon his students the importance of an integrated approach to medicine. What they didn't learn in the classroom, they would master in his busy clinics. It was no accident that he was able to handpick outstanding associates like Haywood and Thomas in the early days of his private practice. His training program at Baylor attracted the best and the brightest; many were already outstanding and experienced pediatricians who self-selected to enhance their training as allergists knowledgeable in the rapidly developing field of immunology.

To work with McGovern in his Texas Medical Center setting was not only to benefit from the clinics, institutions, training programs, and connections throughout the country in the field, but to learn from someone unequalled in his knowledge of the literature being published.

In 1965 McGovern became associate editor of *Annals of Allergy* (now *Annals of Allergy and Immunology*), which during his tenure would become one of the field's leading journals. The *Annals* would be one of twenty-three professional publications at which McGovern would hold editorial appointments during his medical career (see appendix B). The editor, M. Coleman Harris, remembered years later the close attention McGovern had given to editorial work:

> When I assumed editorship of the Annals of Allergy in 1965, Jack became my Associate Editor. It was then that I first became aware of his ability as a medical writer. I found him to be what one would call a thoughtful writer, precise in everything that he put on paper. In utter serenity he writes and rewrites his material until it is perfect, grammatically correct and scientifically sound. He pursues writing with an inner integrity which is impervious to all intrusion from without. Time is of no consequence. On the last occasion we had a conference together it was in the wee hours of the morning before Jack was ready to "call it quits" and go to bed. (I was ready long before then.) Jack is one of the few medical writers I know who weighs each word he puts in writing.[53]

At Baylor McGovern developed an innovative approach for advanced medical training in allergy and immunology, one that is still used today. As a clinical faculty member at Baylor, he also had a founding role in the allergy clinic of Texas Children's Hospital, a newcomer to the Texas Medical Center that opened its doors on February 1, 1954, and is an important story within this story.[54]

Texas Children's Hospital's affiliation with Baylor College of Medicine had begun in 1947 with the appointment of Baylor's first chairman of pediatrics, Russell Blattner (1908–2002). Blattner planned and helped build the Texas Children's Hospital and served as its physician-in-chief. It would become one of the largest children's hospitals in the country and an invaluable resource.

McGovern, as a clinical faculty member of Blattner's Baylor pediatrics department, knew a great deal about running an allergy clinic. So it comes as little surprise that shortly after arriving in Houston and starting his own clinic, McGovern would lend his talents to the new Texas Children's Hospital. McGovern started the allergy clinic there in 1956 in association with the hospital's Junior League Outpatient Department.

Like Osler, who had paid out-of-pocket for microscopes to teach medical students at McGill in the 1870s, McGovern a century later was personally donating supplies and lab equipment from his Montrose clinic to build the fledgling Texas Children's Hospital allergy clinic to serve chronic and severe asthma patients. In time the clinic would become the largest in the hospital's Junior League Outpatient Department and help set Texas Children's Hospital on a trajectory of rapid growth and international recognition.[55]

At McGovern's urging after eighteen years at the helm, on September 1, 1978, the clinic became the Allergy and Immunology Service at Texas Children's. It would have a national reputation that made it possible for Baylor to recruit outstanding talent like William Shearer and David Tanner from St. Louis Children's Hospital—specialists intent on expanding the clinic's capabilities to the next level for treating complex pediatric immunological disorders.[56] Their work would garner headlines read around the world.[57]

One of Shearer's first patients, David Vetter, was a bright and well-informed eight-year-old known as David "the Bubble Boy"—the oldest living child at the time with severe combined immunodeficiency disorder (SCID). Because David lived his life in an isolation bubble, Shearer's search for a solution commanded international attention, even a television documentary.[58] Although David would lose his battle four years later, on February 22, 1984, Shearer and his team learned volumes from the experience, launched aggressive new research programs, and propelled the clinic onto the world stage for unraveling complex regulatory mechanisms of the immune system, including a perplexing newcomer in the early 1980s—AIDS.[59]

THE UT POSTGRADUATE SCHOOL OF MEDICINE

McGovern was also working with Grant Taylor at the University of Texas Postgraduate School of Medicine. The Postgraduate School of Medicine had been handed to Lee Clark by UT's board of regents in 1951, nearly a decade after the creation of the cancer hospital itself in 1942. Its purpose, in the words of the UT regents, was to fulfill the university's "continuing state-wide responsibility for the supervision of the post-degree training of the young physician as an intern and a resident."[60] In hindsight, it was an uphill struggle for Clark. The program lacked support from the medical center and funding from the Texas legislature.[61] From the beginning through the 1950s,[62] funding came primarily through generous gifts from the M. D. Anderson Foundation. Grant Taylor, appointed dean in 1954, was in fact the third dean of the program in forty-eight months (and Mavis Kelsey valiantly served two stints).[63]

In 1963, the Postgraduate School of Medicine was reorganized into two distinct programs: the University of Texas Graduate School of Biomedical Sciences, training PhD researchers in the clinic setting, and the Division of Continuing Medical Education.[64] A history of M. D. Anderson Cancer Center published in 2009 offers a frank assessment:

> The UT Postgraduate School of Medicine had provided an early academic veneer, but many agreed that 'academic appointments for M. D. Anderson did not have sufficient substance in the Postgraduate School.' It never enjoyed the full cooperation of other medical center leaders. Many Baylor faculty believed that the 'Postgraduate School is under the domination of the M. D. Anderson Hospital and might be used to the advantage and disadvantage of some other doctors.' They had resented Clark's appointment as dean, and Grant Taylor's becoming dean in 1954 did nothing to dampen animosities. Convinced that no need existed for a third party to contract residencies and fellowships, other institutions pulled out of the Postgraduate School, which began to hemorrhage.[65]

Taylor saw in McGovern an energetic, natural-born teacher and networker in professional circles who would be ideal to help retool the Postgraduate School into a revitalized continuing education program that would bring Nobel-caliber names in medicine to address Texas Medical Center physicians on timely topics.

In many ways the team of Grant Taylor and Jack McGovern was downright innovative. Recalled Taylor in his memoirs: "Shortly after my arrival in Houston, I learned that the Governor of South Carolina had introduced a novel educational program throughout the State. . . . In essence, the Governor's plan consisted of electronically connecting all of the schools within the State for the purpose of using educational videotapes to enrich the educational curriculum and spare the overburdened teaching corps."

This was a novel idea in the 1960s—to link medical institutions with television for the purpose of continuing education. Today it is, of course, a common concept known as teleconferencing that even a smart phone can handle. For Taylor it was an advance that would expand and revolutionize continuing medical education. But for transformational ideas, sometimes the first steps are the most difficult, as Taylor observed years later:

> In order to simulate the South Carolina system in the Texas Medical Center . . . I arranged for the tape to be transmitted from the University of Texas Dental Branch, and for the signal to go by inter-institutional cable to the M. D. Anderson Hospital and, thence, by a cable which I strung from lamppost to lamppost across the center, then through an open window on the third floor of the library building, and finally, to the projection equipment on the podium in the auditorium of the library building (where the Executive Committee of the Harris County Medical Society eagerly awaited their first look at televised medical education).[66]

As the austere audience assembled, Taylor checked his signal from distant buildings and was greeted with a clear picture that was sure to impress the skeptical crowd. To his dismay, as the meeting was called to order and Taylor took the podium to present this novelty in medical education, a loud "puck" was followed by a blank screen, and the unamazed audience quickly moved to the next item of business.

Taylor would learn that a small transistor costing five cents had shorted out and set medical teleconferencing in Houston back by years. "For the next several years, just as a reminder, I carried the remains of the burned out transistor in my wallet," he would inform all who would listen to his story of a good idea gone bad.

McGovern loved the story and understood clearly how innovations are adopted or delayed by the smallest flaws in planning or the most unexpected events. McGovern's solution was to rehearse and prepare for every possible scenario when presenting new ideas—a commitment to perfection that he practiced repeatedly, often to the distraction of his staff and closest associates.[67]

In time Taylor, with McGovern's input, would help launch a Texas Medical Center television network called UT-TV that today is a highly sophisticated medical television production and teleconferencing program operated by M. D. Anderson Cancer Center—a program now experienced in broadcasting live medical consultations and educational programs worldwide on short notice.

As the fiftieth anniversary of Osler's death on December 29, 1919 approached in 1969, McGovern was hard at work coordinating with the editors of the *Journal of the American Medical Association* (*JAMA*) to prepare a special commemorative issue for December 22, 1969.[68] McGovern and Chuck Roland, a friend and editor at *JAMA*, coordinated more than sixteen essays for the special edition, which went on to inspire the idea of a special symposium under the auspices of the UT Postgraduate School.

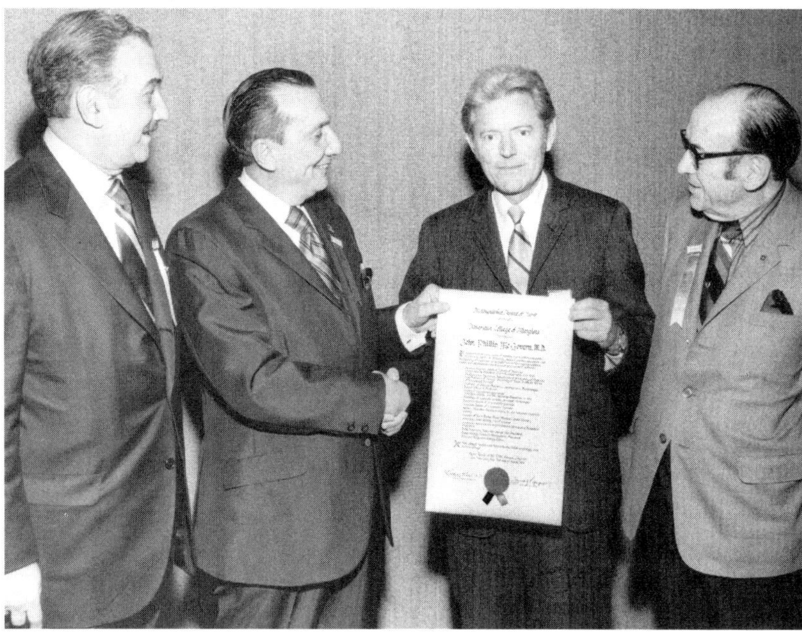

FIGURE 5.6. McGovern receiving the Distinguished Award of Merit from the American College of Allergists in March 1971. Howard G. Rapaport, G. Frederick Hieber, McGovern, Eloi Bauers.

It was to be titled "Humanism in Medicine." McGovern had obtained Davison's blessing for a trial run to determine if enough interest existed across the country to create a professional organization honoring Osler.

When McGovern was installed as president of the American College of Allergists (today known as the American College of Allergy, Asthma and Immunology) in Denver on March 28, 1968, it was a proud moment. With his wife at his side he took the gavel, and his peers across the country gave him their support to lead the profession into new territory as a recognized specialty. The college whose leadership he now took on had been founded in 1942 as McGovern began his medical studies at Duke. Beginning with a membership of a few dozen in the early years of World War II, it has grown to more than five thousand allergists, immunologists, and allied professionals.

During his presidential year of 1968–1969 McGovern addressed a variety of complex issues, but none were more difficult than the struggle for an independent American Board of Allergy. If Mac had been alive, he would no doubt have been reminded by his son's national leadership of his own years of service on behalf of the medical profession at the DC Medical Society. Without his father to confide in, McGovern turned to Dean Davison to share his challenges and strategies. "As you may know," he wrote Davison on August 8, 1968,

> the allergists have been "fighting" for 25 years for an independent American Board of Allergy. I'm not certain whether this is good or bad but, at any rate, at the Allergy Section of the AMA meeting in June, with the approval by vote of the American College of Allergists and the American Academy of Allergy against a coalition of the so-called "non-Boarded allergists" (actually not sub-Boarded), we passed the Sherman Resolution for an independent board and sent it on [to] the Advisory Board for the Medical Specialties. They will act on it in February. An editorial which relates to this is enclosed—not particularly well written but I did have the temerity of quoting Osler, and thus thought that you might like to read it. It seems that during most of these battles one hardly ever hears of the patient's welfare being considered.[69]

McGovern's year as president culminated in the organization's April 1969 annual meeting in Washington, DC, featuring a guest presentation by Sir William Osler's student Wilburt Davison.

Orville Thomas and Theodore Haywood, senior associates from McGovern's Houston clinic, rushed a co-signed message back to the staff in Houston as the meeting closed, announcing that McGovern had eloquently introduced Davison to an audience of a thousand and that Davison's speech had been "the finest and most heart-warming . . . that we have ever had the pleasure of hearing." They added that McGovern during his presidential address had had no fewer than three standing ovations. "It was by far the best meeting of the College during the 25 years that it has been in existence."[70]

The first of McGovern's honorary doctoral degrees came in 1971 from Ricker College, a small college within the University of Maine System. In time twenty-eight other universities, including Kent State, the University of Nebraska, Florida State, and his own Duke University, would award honorary doctorates for his academic and civic contributions.

During the 1970s McGovern's name was becoming widely known in national medical circles. His allergy clinic, training programs in allergy/immunology, editorial roles with a growing number of professional journals, published professional articles and books, innovative and popular continuing education programs, and rapidly growing foundation were collectively making him a name few could ignore in medical—or

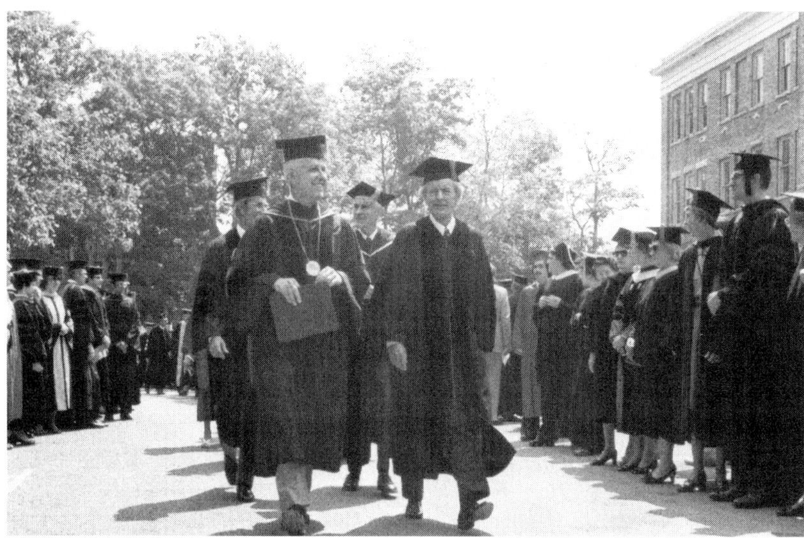

FIGURE 5.7. McGovern (front right) at Ball State University to receive one of his twenty-nine honorary doctorates. President John Prius (front left) leads the procession on commencement day, May 20, 1977.

business—circles. Dean Davison took special notice of his prize student from Duke days when he learned that even the president of the United States had taken notice. "Needless to say," he wrote McGovern, "I was delighted that you have been appointed by Mr. Nixon as a member of the Board of Regents of the National Library of Medicine. Not only is it a very distinguished Board, but it is actually getting things accomplished through the Public Health Service which those of us who were on the previous Board could not get done through the Army."[71]

Houston, a city built on Texas-sized ideas, certainly had its share of medical giants and financial success stories—but never had it had someone like Jack McGovern, who was a name to watch in both spheres.

Don't Call Me Philanthropist

Jack McGovern did not like being called a philanthropist. He was a physician, scientist, and medical educator first and foremost. It was as such that he wanted to be known, and to his mind his reputation as a philanthropist was a distraction that should not be allowed to overshadow his medical contributions as a physician. The very sound of the word philanthropist would draw his silent displeasure. He saw building a foundation and giving away millions of dollars to his profession and his community as just a sidebar to his medical career. Yet the success of his investments and the dramatic growth of the John P. McGovern Foundation over time made it very difficult to maintain the quiet, low-key civic image he continuously sought.

Early on he did not put his name on the foundation; but as his philanthropy built on his medical career, so his medical career built on his philanthropy. He was who he was and was able to do what he did in part because people knew his name. And so eventually it found its way into the name of the foundation and onto public libraries, zoos, medical museums and buildings, endowed lectureships and professorships, and teaching awards throughout the country (see appendix C).

This reluctance about philanthropy was never a question of McGovern's wanting to hide his light under a bushel; it was a question of where exactly he wanted it to shine, and he wanted it to shine on his medical career. But his preference not to be called a philanthropist was ultimately unachievable, and in the end, he surrendered to reality and even enjoyed it. In his heart of hearts, however, he was always a physician first.

He would be honored time and time again in later life for his generous gifts and humanitarian spirit. It is through the gifts of his foundation that he will always be remembered, medical career aside, for generosity.[72] For that reason, the narrative of his foundation and his outlook on giving is a defining story within his lifetime of stories.

From the day in 1961 when McGovern started his foundation with $10,000, he worked with the same intensity and drive on the business side of his life as he did on his medical career.

Even in childhood, McGovern had understood that to have resources was better than not to have them, and that options not only for enjoying life but also for helping other people enjoy it increased dramatically with means at hand. He had seen the pleasure his cousin Helen Hayes had experienced in creating her foundation and giving to the arts. Through her connections and fame, she had been able to open doors and help people on a scale that was truly enviable.

And then there was Davison, who had informed his young protégé that, with the exception of his time in the army, he had always managed to live off income earned through investments and book sales, never depending on his paycheck from work.[73] Davison's letters to McGovern over the years mentioned sales of his textbook (meticulously recorded as $92,464.32)[74] along with occasional stock investments ($6,000 annual income at retirement)[75] that clearly sent a message: building outside income for retirement was not to be overlooked. For McGovern this was not new information, but a reinforcement of lessons he had learned from his Granny Brown, who had memorably introduced him to the idea of investing his first $7 in a bank to earn interest. Over the years McGovern fine-tuned his skills at saving and investing in ways that his family and Wilburt Davison never imagined.

And Granny Brown, who had been so openhanded during the Depression, had also given another important lesson in giving: she never asked anything in return for what she gave, McGovern would recall years later. She understood that the gift of giving brought a personal reward that had nothing to do with material value. McGovern best summarized her outlook in 1996 to *Houston Chronicle* reporter Shelby Hodge: "I learned from watching my grandmother that giving and receiving is the same thing. I could see in her eyes that it made her feel good. It helped her soul when she was giving."[76]

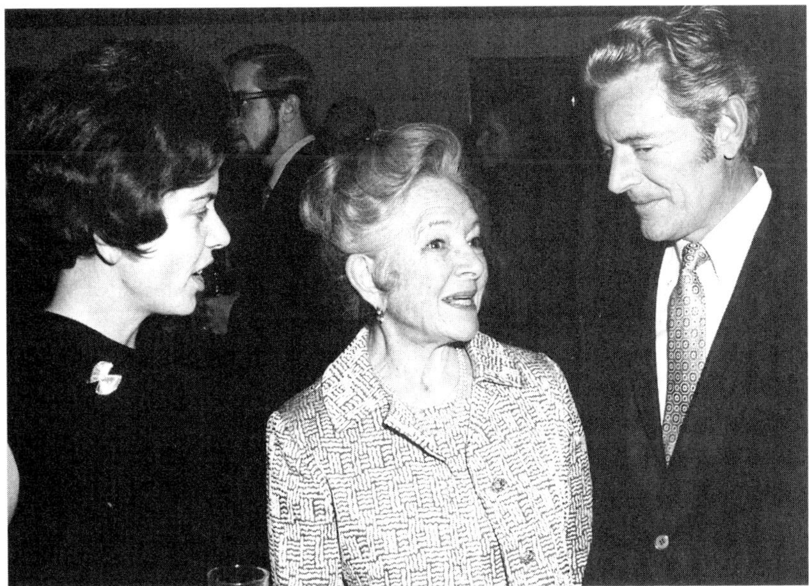

FIGURE 5.8. Helen Hayes flanked by second cousin McGovern and Kathy.

McGovern's fund was one that he never stopped building. When TARF was renamed the John P. McGovern Foundation in 1979, it would have a broader mandate to allow gifts to support the medical community as well as civic causes such as zoos and libraries to benefit children and families. As the original $10,000 grew into millions, McGovern's investment career filled every spare moment not occupied by his medical career—or fishing.

Kathy was a silent partner with little direct involvement in her husband's investments. But she had always supported them, from the early days of their marriage when she had driven him around Houston neighborhoods in search of properties to buy. And she had watched with some astonishment as his successes in business snowballed. After his death in 2007, she would comfortably assume his role as president of the foundation, and she now runs the foundation she watched him build.

By day McGovern saw patients and oversaw his successful clinic enterprise and medical career. By night and on weekends he searched for opportunities to invest in real estate and the stock market.

Kathy, who knew him best, nevertheless remains lost for words to identify the source of McGovern's talent for business deals and investing.

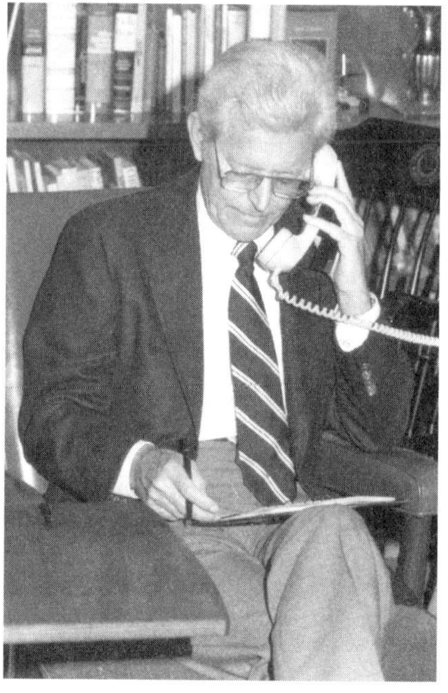
Figure 5.9. McGovern in the 1980s.

It was a talent that coupled with his intense drive and nonstop energy made him an investment success. His father, a surgeon, instilled in him a moral sense of helping others, but his father did not make a lot of money at all and did not give him such a business head. No, he didn't get that from his father; I don't really know where he got it. I think it's all his own . . . I am certain that Jack could have been the CEO of any Fortune 500 company in this country, without question, if he had not chosen medicine as his first priority.

I can tell you his investment career started about the time we were married in the early 1960s. He did not like to drive a car, he liked to think and talk. So I was his chauffeur, and we went all over the neighborhood over there by the Texas Medical Center and Shamrock Hotel, and he started picking up property and putting it together. He just loved negotiating and making deals and driving around after work looking for property that would connect to property he owned. In time, investment groups he came to know and trust offered opportunities for him to invest. In that way he purchased the Brompton property his clinic was built on in the 1970s.[77]

As the foundation grew through the 1970s and 1980s, McGovern added real estate tax advisors, accountants, and legal representation. Orville Story (1925–2012) first joined McGovern in 1972 as a tax-planning advisor on a short-term contract that was originally set for three months, but lasted forty years. It was McGovern's CPA, Al Kramer, who first suggested that Story and McGovern should meet. Story would, in time, serve as director and treasurer of the foundation and a member of the board of directors until his sudden death from a stroke on May 27, 2012.[78] Just two years before his death he reflected on his years working with McGovern.

> I called Dr. McGovern and we had a short interview on the telephone and he asked me to come talk to him. I think it was three months before the end of the year. And so he got somebody and drew up a contract for us that I'm not sure was ever signed. The next thing I know, a year had gone by. We just never discussed another contract and never discussed much of anything but working. We never had a formal agreement. I just kept working and he kept giving me more work. I had an office in a separate office building, and eventually he asked me to move to his new building and work permanently for him and no one else. . . .
>
> I can tell you we just had work piled up so much that there wasn't anybody else I could work for. We did seem to be able to communicate with each other, and I worked specifically in the business area, not the medical side. There were some unique opportunities to own real estate with some tax planning, and that was where most of our work was going. However, the real estate turned out to be not only tax planning but good investments.
>
> Dr. McGovern's ability to view things was far ahead of other people that I had ever seen or worked with. One of his unique things was his ability to understand timing. He used timing to absolutely the ultimate in having investments being profitable. I happen to have known his stock broker, who said to me that Dr. McGovern's ability to understand the value of different securities was far greater than any other client that he had, and from time to time the home office in New York would call their Houston office and ask, "What is Dr. McGovern doing?," which was a good observation by them.
>
> He had an ability to understand real estate. His ability to understand was so broad and so superior to other people it was unreal. It made it very difficult to work with him from time to time, but he seemed to understand the growth pattern of the city of Houston, and which real estate had the most opportunity for increasing in value. His style was to buy property and almost never sell it.[79]

In fact, Story said, McGovern sold real estate only when demand was at its peak and then only to its "end-user"—which is to say, for the highest price it could possibly bring.

McGovern had a gift for seeing the big picture and an innate ability to predict the trends and understand the equilibrium of markets. The health of financial markets and portfolios requires a broad perspective and an extraordinary sense of timing—timing that McGovern had in spades. Much as his work as a physician/scientist relied on making informed decisions based on patient data, his investment strategies were informed by market data that he meticulously kept in a small black book—strategies that if studied carefully should be replicable. Story knew McGovern's strategies well.

> He was proud of this little black book where he would keep his record of stocks that he wanted to buy. He was a very busy man as he donated all of his time to the medical practice during the day, and would work on his stocks at night and on weekends. And particularly on weekends, we would review all of the portfolios that he had and what he wanted to add and the new ones that he may have decided because of the style of the stock or the area of the market that he wanted to get into. . . . I read those little numbers so much my eyes would blink. So I had to give him high and low and a medium—some middle ground—on some. But that was how he made his decisions. He would make notes, and then after we would finish, he would normally call his broker on Sunday night and give the sell or buy orders.[80]

While the McGovern Foundation portfolio continued to grow—well diversified across stocks, bonds, precious metals, and real estate—it was the real estate investments that kept Story busy around the clock.

> Well, the interesting thing is, every time he went somewhere his interest was looking at real estate. If he'd go to California, for example, he would look at the different markets and the ones that had the upside like in a condo or apartment project. My function was that he would call me if he got involved in buying in another city. I would go to California and work with the real estate brokers and help him with his negotiating style with the brokers. And we bought property in California and in Florida, some in Tennessee, and other valuable places in the country—well, I guess we were limited more to those three states. And I use 'we' loosely as it was all him, I was just part of the team.
>
> He worked hard and was very frugal in his lifestyle. He was very closed about his investments and did not like to be noted as an investor or philanthropist as he wanted to be noted as the physician at the top of his field

> that he was. I would say he coupled his sense of timing with investments that were solid and never risky. He was never interested in a fancy proposal by anybody. He felt like anytime that there was a proposal that was tied up in a ribbon or something, he did not need to look at that. He only wanted to look at maybe one or two sheets of something that was proposed and just see the facts of it.[81]

Working with the same drive and passion that built his medical career and clinic, McGovern grew his foundation through relentless attention to his black book and the opportunities at hand. The same attention that went into investing he also put into the distribution of foundation funds. Typically at least 5 percent of the previous year's average net assets are required by the IRS to be distributed for charitable purposes.

Settling into a familiar routine, he would work with his staff daily to review requests and opportunities for good causes that sought his approval. His attention to every detail and dollar was in keeping with his frugal nature. For example, a $200 printer that did not seem necessary, buried in the budget of an otherwise good proposal requesting $5,000, might provoke a prolonged discussion analyzing and reanalyzing the motivation and justification for that one item before McGovern would approve a check for $4,800 . . . or reject the proposal outright.

In the spring of 1981 the leaders of the Texas Medical Center did something never done before when they organized a testimonial dinner in McGovern's honor. For the first time in the history of the Texas Medical Center, all of the presidents of each institution combined their efforts to honor one individual. Orville Thomas, in attendance that evening, was so impressed that he summarized his impressions in a letter he sent to a long list of McGovern's colleagues and former students, noting, "I can not begin to describe the magnificent accolades that were heaped on Jack during the dinner ceremony. . . . Leon Jaworski was absolutely great in his 20 minute speech about Jack—better than I've ever heard him locally or on national television."[82]

Among the institutional leaders honoring McGovern that night along with Leon Jaworski, chairman of the Texas Medical Center's board of directors, was Roger J. Bulger, president of the University of Texas Health Science Center at Houston (1978–1987). The chief administrator of six professional schools including medicine, public health, dentistry, and nursing, Bulger remembers having been given strong support by McGovern, who,

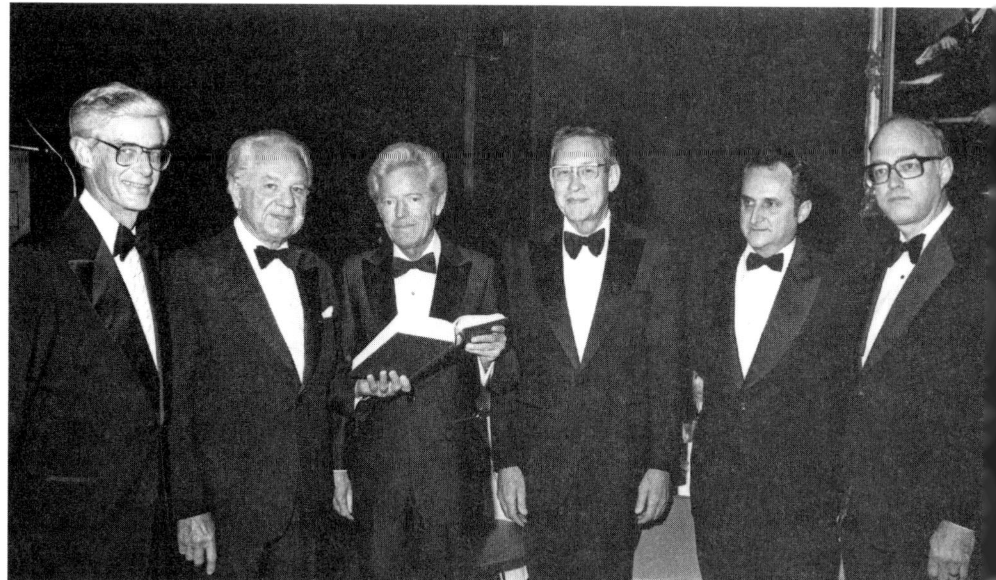

FIGURE 5.10. Texas Medical Center leaders honor McGovern in a one-of-a-kind recognition ceremony on May 5, 1981. L-R, Charles LeMaistre (president, MD Anderson System Cancer Center), Leon Jaworski (president, Texas Medical Center Board), McGovern, Jack Williams (Executive Director, Texas Medical Center), Roger J. Bulger (president, University of Texas Health Science Center at Houston), and William T. Butler (president, Baylor College of Medicine).

he says, "invested in me as an administrator championing his firm belief that leadership of large academic health care institutions should be committed to humanistic and Hippocratic values in the training of individual physicians as well as health care teams."[83]

Bulger would leave Houston and the Texas Medical Center to become the president of the Association of Academic Health Centers in Washington, DC, for nearly two decades (1988–2005). Thus he has both a Houston-based and a national perspective on McGovern's work. At the national level, he recalls, he came to fully appreciate McGovern's reach beyond Houston and the Texas Medical Center. He remembers that he felt a sense of pride (and often surprise) each time he discovered another McGovern-supported national or international initiative he had not known of. He found that McGovern worked tirelessly nationally as well as locally with academic leaders. He collaborated on publications[84] and championed national conferences related to the medical humanities and ethics.

Bulger adds that McGovern helped administrators in many ways that went beyond supporting their programs with endowments and other financial means. He provided his insights into the relevance of human values to the art of medicine—in short, he shared his vision. And with it he gave inspiration to those in positions of power to keep health care moving toward a more sensitive humanitarianism even as it moved toward a better science. Bulger's book, *Healing America,* published in 2010, addresses "the healing *relationship* [my italics] that can occur between patients and health care professionals."[85] The first person cited on the book's dedication page—John P. McGovern.

McGovern focused much of his energy on programs directed toward the prevention of disease—"to address what I call the diseases of lifestyle, each one of which has an addictive nature."[86] This included programs aimed at preventing heart disease and its determinants, including smoking, alcohol, and obesity. Even as an undergraduate at Duke, McGovern had shown an

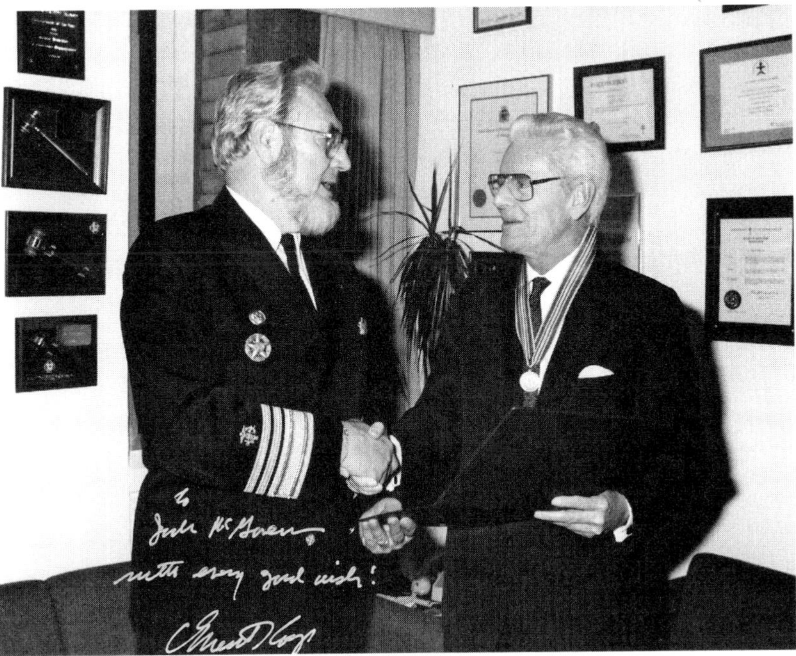

FIGURE 5.11. McGovern and Surgeon General C. Everett Koop in April 1984. McGovern was receiving the Surgeon General's Medallion for his work in alcoholism and drug abuse.

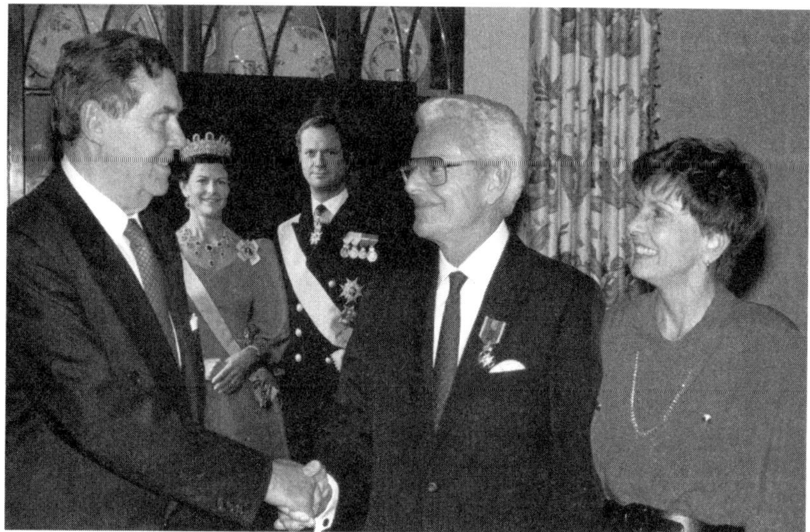

FIGURE 5.12. McGovern received the Swedish Royal Medallion of the Polar Star, awarded in Houston in 1988. Kathy is beside him; a portrait of King Carl XVI Gustaf and Queen Silvia is in the background.

interest in the health effects of addictions, as his concerned letters home, cited previously, indicate—"Have you given up smoking again father, have you quit drinking?"[87] In the spring of 1940 he wrote a theme titled "The Psychological Aspects of Drug Addiction." Reporting on it in a letter to his mother, he said, "If I ever get into Public Health work, the knowledge I have gained from research on this paper will stand me in good stead."[88] And in fact nearly fifty years later, in April 1989, McGovern was in Washington to receive the Surgeon General Medallion presented by C. Everett Koop for his leadership (both as a physician and as a businessman) in preventing alcoholism and drug abuse.

The Surgeon General was not the only Washington official taking notice of McGovern. Over in the White House, President Ronald Reagan had on his desk nominations for McGovern to receive the Presidential Medal of Freedom, the nation's highest civilian honor.[89] But McGovern, an active Republican throughout his professional life, was never to receive that medal despite repeated nominations, including one in 1991 directed to President George H. Bush by Betty Ford.[90]

Six years earlier, in 1985, McGovern had received the Private Sector Initiative Commendation from President Reagan, only to be overshadowed a year later when his cousin Helen received the more prestigious Presidential Medal of Freedom. Perhaps this friendly competition with his famous cousin intensified McGovern's investment of time and resources for the community good, as by 1988 his foundation was now valued at over $50 million and was growing rapidly.[91]

One of McGovern's favorite responses when asked about his foundation and his gifts was, "It's all about feeling good inside. I think everybody's got an empty spot inside, and I call it the God-sized hole that we have to fill. And you can't do that with Caesar's-world stuff—money, property, prestige. That doesn't fill that hole. Love does . . . Love in the sense of deep caring."[92]

And always, when his accomplishments in medicine were compared with his accomplishments in investments and giving, his first thought was—just don't call me philanthropist.

Chapter Six

Legacies

Renaissance Man

On the evening of September 13, 2001, just two days after the fall of the twin towers in New York City, Houston stopped for a brief moment to honor John P. McGovern in an extraordinary way. On that night more than twelve hundred Houstonians, including the mayor and state and nationally elected officials, gathered in the Imperial Ballroom of Houston's Hyatt Regency to put aside the national turmoil and celebrate McGovern as Houston's Distinguished Citizen of the Year.[1]

Former president George H. W. Bush and his wife Barbara, both community-invested Houstonians, were honorary chairs for the evening. They set aside the international crisis that their son in the White House was handling to send a videotaped message of appreciation. All eyes were on the ballroom's big screen as former president Bush ("41" in presidential shorthand) addressed the man of the hour:

> It is my pleasure to join you in recognizing the Rotary Club of Houston's Distinguished Citizen of 2001. As a child of the depression, tonight's honoree learned from his parents that the needs of people come first and that monetary rewards are really secondary. While growing up in Washington, DC, during that dark period in our history, he saw how his father, the surgeon, was usually 'the last to be paid.' He learned from this special role model that giving and receiving are the same thing.

> . . . This individual followed in his father's footsteps with a love for medicine and a deep commitment to helping humankind. Besides the zoo and Houston's parks, he is a major contributor to our museums, the Texas Medical Center and many, many other important causes. The list could go on, and should include the fact that he has devoted his medical career to battling such common ills as those caused by pollen and ragweed. He founded the McGovern Allergy Clinic, the largest private allergy clinic in the nation. . . . Thank you, Jack, for serving as an example to your community, your city, and your country, as our new Distinguished Citizen. I wish you and Kathy all the very best.[2]

Charles A. LeMaistre, former chancellor of the University of Texas System (1971–1978) and the successor to Lee Clark as president of M. D. Anderson Cancer Center (1978–1996), added this to the accolades:

> In these turbulent days, when freedom and civility are once again under attack by barbarians, we must remember the greatness of a nation is not measured solely by its tall buildings, its military power, or its wealth, but primarily by the qualities of the citizen it produces. . . . Dr. Jack McGovern is a unique, humane and gifted leader—who displays talents and interests in such breadth and of such diversity—to deserve the appellation, 'A Modern Day Renaissance Man.'[3]

During the last decade of his life McGovern rarely accepted awards in person, but that night was something different, and he ascended the podium with the careful gait and concentration of a man three months into his ninth decade. The words of his allotted ten minutes were carefully crafted. When you gave Jack McGovern ten minutes for remarks, you got exactly ten minutes—not a minute more or less.

Accepting praise was difficult for McGovern, no matter how much practice he had doing it, and this was especially true in retirement; he preferred during his final years to remain low-key and out of the public spotlight. These would be the last public remarks he would make before his death six years later. His mission that night was to deflect the spotlight from himself to those he credited with his success in life:

> It is with great pleasure that I accept the distinguished citizen award this evening. . . . I want to thank someone very special. Without her I doubt I would even be alive, much less here tonight to enjoy this event. I want to thank my dearest wife of forty years, Kathy. I must admit that I have had great, loving role models since birth and much help and support along the way before arriving at this podium tonight. My mother, father, grandmother, aunts and uncles were wonderful, powerful models of unconditional love and moral values by words and deeds. From them I learned a way of life. Enough cannot be said about the importance of role models and those who influence you in powerful ways without even knowing it.
>
> . . . I have had one key mentor and lifelong friend in my medical years whom I think about every day since his death in 1972, Dr. Wilburt C. Davison. . . . His positive example as a physician/scientist, a humane person who cared deeply about his patients and students will never be forgotten. Dean Davison taught by example and made a difference in many lives, including that of John P. McGovern. I gladly accept this award with each and every one of these individuals in mind who have influenced and helped me along the way.[4]

McGovern was aware that this night was an exceptional community acknowledgement of his lifework. He had set out to do great things, and he had done them. The standing ovation from the audience provided a thunderous stamp of approval that surely would have also brought to their feet Mac, Lottie, Granny Brown, Helen, Dean Davison, and all the others McGovern had cared about and prized during his lifetime. Perhaps even Osler himself would have been moved to stand in applause.

The three selected stories that follow exemplify the legacy that was honored that night and that reaches far beyond Houston and the Texas Medical Center. If McGovern could direct the order of these three stories, without question he would start with Osler.

Honoring Osler—The American Osler Society

Step forward a decade in time from this award ceremony. Nearly four years have passed since McGovern's death in May 2007. It is May 1, 2011, and the forty-first annual meeting of the American Osler Society has brought to the city of Philadelphia 132 medical historians and scholars who share a common interest in Sir William Osler and the history of medicine.[5]

While the society is small for an international organization, those accepted into its membership are respected medical historians, predominantly physicians who share a common passion for the ideals Sir William Osler modeled more than a century before. During the next three days, these members will present sixty-five papers.[6] The scholars of the history of medicine who are in attendance and presenting the papers represent many of the most prestigious medical universities in the United States, Canada, Great Britain, and Japan. They will compare notes on academic programs that improve the training of physicians, spotlight the importance of the humanities to medicine, and encourage the mix of art and science that the profession benefits from so profoundly, yet often loses sight of.

In 2011, forty-one years after McGovern helped launch the Osler Society, he is no longer there to present papers and network with colleagues, but his presence is still felt. The John P. McGovern Lecture is an annual centerpiece of the meeting, and the selected speaker's presentation is always reprinted and widely distributed. For the first time in the organization's history, the number of papers to be presented requires concurrent sessions to fit everything (including special presentations by medical students who will be the next generation of medical historians) into the three-day calendar.

On the third day of the meeting an elderly man, legally blind and confined to a wheelchair, is escorted by his daughter to a spot in the back of the room. He sits forward, listening intently to the presentations as his colleagues of the past, and new ones he has never met, go about the business of scholarship. His name is Alfred Henderson, and he is a charter member of the American Osler Society.

Henderson and McGovern met in 1967 and discussed their common interest in creating a professional organization to honor the ideals of Sir William Osler. Chief among those was the belief that "the practice of medicine requires knowledge and skill, frequently labeled as the science and art of medicine," as McGovern would write in *Humanism in Medicine.*[7] But in the late 1960s, McGovern was brooding over a concern he harbored that the medical profession was focused too much on the science and too little on the art. Osler had exemplified both, and his ideals were in jeopardy if physicians of the future did not use heart as well as head to provide the care patients needed. The combination of science and art best assured that the practice of medicine would remain a profession and not devolve into trade

In the fall of 1967 McGovern had no idea who Alfred Henderson was or that the two would soon join forces to create the American Osler Society. But Henderson, a physician and a consultant to the Division of Medical Science at the Smithsonian, shared McGovern's interest in Osler's ideas. And, while McGovern and Henderson did not know each other, Wilburt Davison knew them both; and he was the catalyst who brought the two like minds together. In a letter dated October 9, 1967, he told McGovern, "I have written to Dr. Alfred R. Henderson of the Division of Medicine of the Smithsonian Institute that you were a fellow Oslerian and that you would call on him the next time you are in Washington."[8] McGovern was in Washington within weeks to attend a medical meeting, and he followed up on the obligation Davison had put him under.

His first meeting with Henderson was the beginning of a relationship based on a mutual commitment to create an organization dedicated to Osler. And it was memorable partly because it involved George Washington's false teeth. Davison, at his country home in the Blue Ridge Mountains seventy-six miles from Durham, received a letter from McGovern dated October 31:

> Kathy and I just returned yesterday from our meeting in Washington where I gave two papers. May I thank you so very much for inscribing the pictures that we took in Roaring Gap and particularly for the one of you and William Osler.
>
> Thanks to your letter of introduction, the highlight of our trip to Washington was a delightful visit with Dr. Alfred Henderson. He spent the better part of an afternoon with me and we talked of Davison and Osler to our hearts' content. He showed me all around the medical exhibits at the Smithsonian and in his office and let me hold George Washington's false teeth, saying that "Yours are the last hands to hold these before they go on permanent exhibit next Monday."
>
> Dr. Henderson told me of his plans and some of his problems concerning them. I believe that I might be able to be of some help in some way. Also, he discussed the organization of an "International Osler Society" and we also plan to write an article together.[9]

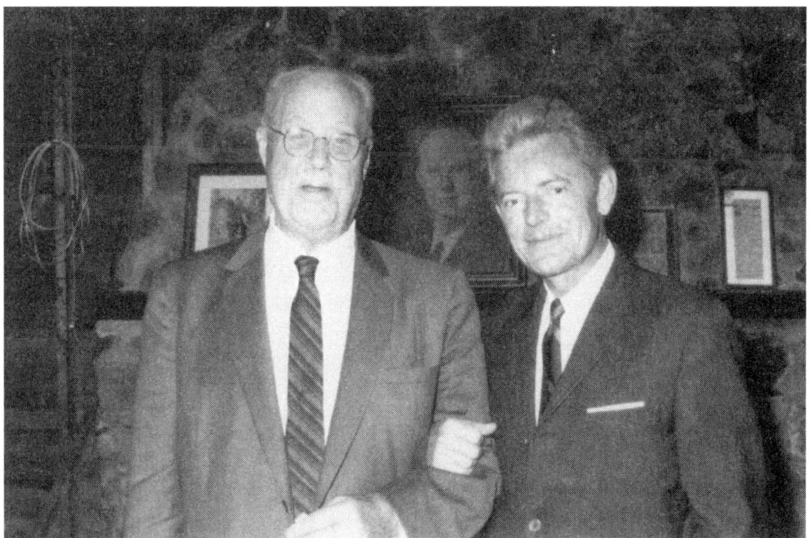

FIGURE 6.1. McGovern arm-in-arm with Wilburt Davison at Davison's home in Roaring Gap, North Carolina, in 1968. Photo by Kathy McGovern.

Shortly after that first meeting the two went to work to canvass medical professionals in the United States and Canada who were well known for their interest in Osler. McGovern posed the possibility of an Osler society's forming as a "rumor" going around, an interesting technique that he was known to use from time to time in order to appear neutral as he indirectly tested the waters when fishing for support. In fact, Davison was one of the fish he caught:

December 1, 1969
Dear Jack:

I enjoyed our telephone conversation this morning. I also have heard rumors of the formation of an American Osler Society, and I hope very much that one can be formed. Osler's influence is more needed today than ever before.

Atala joins me in love to Kathy and you.
Yours affectionately,
Dave.[10]

Henderson and McGovern drafted a statement of purpose, designed a logo,[11] arranged for printing of membership certificates and programs, and established a temporary board.[12]

It was during these formative years of the new organization that McGovern, never one to miss an opportunity, approached the editorial staff of the *Journal of the American Medical Association* with the idea of publishing a special issue of *JAMA* in December 1969 to commemorate the fiftieth anniversary of Osler's death.[13] He collaborated on the project with Charles Roland (1933–2009), a physician and a member of *JAMA*'s editorial staff. The successful Osler issue led to future collaborations with Roland, who would become an early member of the Osler Society and a historian of the organization.[14]

While McGovern would have been delighted to see Davison president of the Osler Society, Davison, now seventy-nine, flatly rejected the idea, insisting that the organization needed a younger leader. William B. Bean (1909–1989), the Sir William Osler Professor of Medicine at Iowa City, was quickly identified as the right man for the job. Bean, who headed the Department of Internal Medicine at the University of Iowa College of Medicine, had first learned of Osler as a child when his father, a physician, brought home both volumes of Cushing's Pulitzer Prize-winning biography of Osler. "As was his custom, he began reading page 1, chapter 1, vol. 1, aloud to the family," Bean wrote later. "Along about the middle of it, . . . I got so interested that I picked up vol. 2 and read that through before Father had finished vol. 1. . . . I remember being totally desolate when I read about Revere's death in France and Osler's heroic, but profoundly depressive, reaction after his bereavement."[15]

Charles Roland, writing in his historical overview of the Osler Society (2002), chronicled classic McGovern, who was not to be deflected, however briefly, in his quest to secure Bean's agreement to serve as president of the new organization. "On Sunday 30 November 1969," he records, "Jack McGovern called Iowa City and traced Bean to Clinton, Iowa, and to—not surprisingly—a tennis court. A call to the clubhouse brought Bill breathlessly away from his game. Jack explained what was happening, because at this stage Bean was unaware the society was being created. McGovern extended the invitation, Bean accepted, and returned to finish his set."[16]

An initial letter inviting charter members was distributed by McGovern within days of Bean's agreement to lead the organization. Interestingly, McGovern gives the appearance of distancing himself from direct involvement in shaping the organization. This is the content of the letter:

> Al Henderson, one of the Curators for Medicine at the Smithsonian, and a number of other Oslerians around the nation have decided to organize the American Osler Society. . . . The thought immediately came to my mind that you might be interested in joining this organization. As I understand it, a brief statement of its purposes would be documented essentially as follows:
>
> The purpose of the Society is to unite, into an organized group, physicians, and others allied to the profession, with a common interest in memorializing and perpetuating the lessons of the life and teachings of William Osler; to meet periodically for the purpose of presentation and discussion of papers on the life and influence of Osler upon the profession, and to publish these essays as a Proceeding of the Society; to continually place before the profession a reminder of the high principles of life and humanism in the practice of Osler, and to introduce these things to those entering the profession.
>
> Membership in this organization will be limited to real Oslerians who have published something on or about Osler and who have demonstrated significant interest in Osleriana. The two living Rhodes Scholars under Osler, namely, Wilburt Cornell Davison, Dean Emeritus of Duke, and Wilder Penfield, have both lent their support to this organization and will be elected Honorary Members. Although there are many student Osler Clubs around the country, it is felt that an organization such as this can help to stimulate humanism in medicine as expressed by the life and work of William Osler at a time when it is sorely needed.
>
> The dues in this organization will be minimal, as I understand it, and the secretary would be able to let you know of this at a later date. Please let me know of your interest at your earliest convenience.[17]

From Houston, McGovern worked by telephone and through personal letters to arrange for incorporation of the new organization and a first meeting at the Flagship Hotel in Galveston in April 1970.[18] He had the help of Grant Taylor, now overseeing the restructured continuing-education role of the UT Postgraduate School of Medicine, and colleagues Truman Blocker and Chester Burns at the UT Medical Branch in Galveston.

The Galveston symposium further confirmed that there was enough interest to merit creating a professional organization in Osler's name. The meeting was well attended and supportive. Its proceedings generated

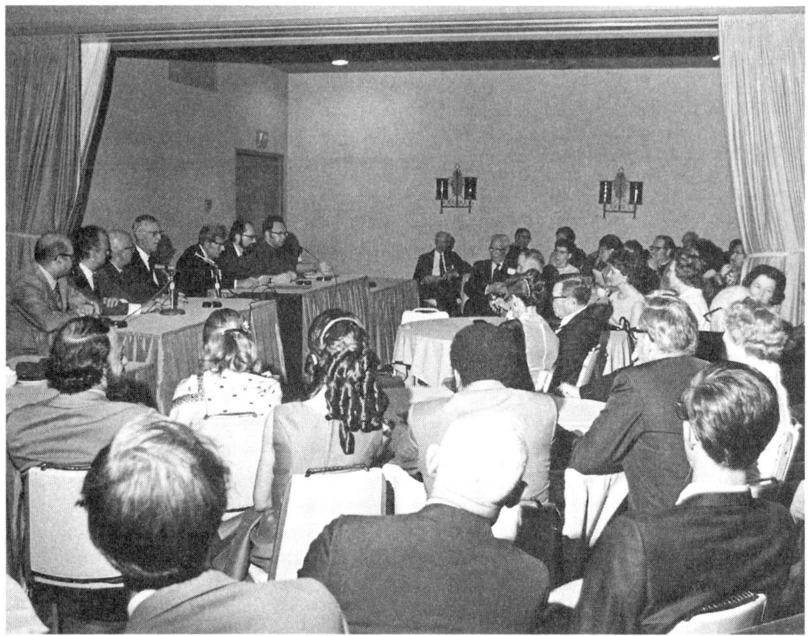

FIGURE 6.2. The Flagship Hotel in Galveston was the site of an April 1970 symposium on humanism and medicine. It served as a test run for launching the American Osler Society.

McGovern and Burns's *Humanism in Medicine* and set the stage for the organization's first annual meeting, slated for the following year in Denver.[19]

Henderson's introductory remarks at the first annual meeting in Denver on April 1, 1971, spoke directly to an issue close to McGovern's heart:

> One of the chief legacies of William Osler is the concept, reiterated time and again to his students and young practitioners, that the practice of medicine consists of much more than the science of preserving health, curing diseases and prolonging life. The heritage of Osler contains the admonition that science is but a part of practice and that the real need of the profession at large is the quality of humanism and the mark of the cultured gentleman. . . . It is a sad and serious observation that far too many twentieth century physicians are concerned chiefly with the science and economics of medicine. Witness the all-too-common 'pay when served' signs that confront those who enter the waiting rooms of our colleagues, transmuting instantly what we must respectfully call a 'patient' into a 'client.'[20]

Such is the way McGovern and Henderson took a common idea, settled on a plan of action, assimilated like minds, and founded an organization that continues to this day to fulfill an important scholarly need.

McGovern never wanted credit as founder of the Osler Society. He understood that such undertakings resulted, as Charles Roland pointed out, from a "zeitgeist"—a pattern of thought or feeling characteristic of a time.[21] The American Osler Society emerged in large part from the mid-century sense that medicine was in danger of losing the blend of art with science that is essential to the physician's calling: "Twin berries on one stem," Osler called them. "Grievous damage has been done to both in regarding the Humanities and Science in any other light than complemental."[22] Many people in medical education share that view today and a growing number of medical humanities programs at medical schools across the country now address the issue. Such programs complement the science of medicine with the art of medicine in order to produce well-rounded new physicians who embrace the old traditions that Osler embodied.[23]

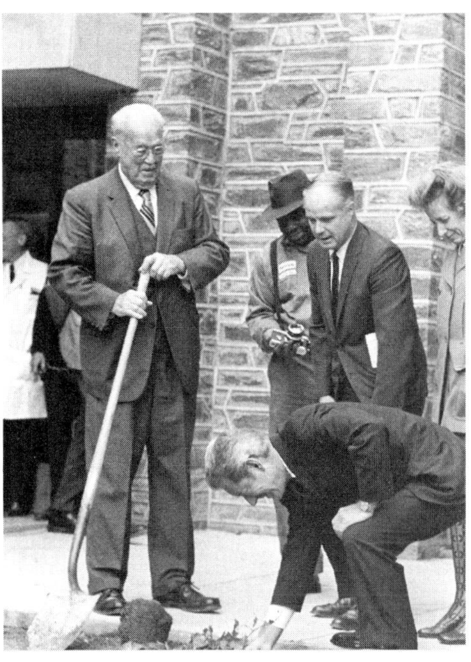

FIGURE 6.3. Duke, 1969. McGovern plants a sprig of ivy from Osler's Oxford home. Davison standing at left, Al Henderson behind McGovern.

Two such programs share McGovern's name: the McGovern Center for Humanities and Ethics at the UT Health Science Center at Houston[24] (where he held faculty appointments at each of the institution's six schools and was the only faculty member with that distinction) and the John P. McGovern Academy of Oslerian Medicine at the UT Medical Branch at Galveston.[25]

In 2011, as an elderly Al Henderson sat in his wheelchair in the back of the crowded Philadelphia auditorium listening to the proceedings of the Osler Society's forty-first annual assembly, he must surely have remembered that first meeting with his then newfound friend Jack McGovern—a meeting at which George Washington's false teeth were in attendance as plans for honoring Osler began to cohere.

From Index Catalog to PubMed—The National Library of Medicine

The National Library of Medicine rose from a small post-Civil War collection of medical books to become a national treasure. It is now the world's largest collection of biomedical literature. To serve on its board of regents requires presidential appointment. Established in 1956, the sixteen-member board meets three times a year and serves in an advisory capacity to the secretary of health and human services on all matters affecting the library.[26]

In a handwritten letter dated January 23, 1970, the library's director, Martin Cummings (1920–2011), informed McGovern that "today I nominated you to serve as a member of the National Library of Medicine Board of Regents. The process is long and arduous but I hope the President and the Senate will accept my nomination because you will be a great asset to us as a steward and friend of libraries and scholarship."[27] In October of the same year, President Richard Nixon approved the nomination.

For someone like McGovern—who loved medical history, collected rare books and medallions, valued scholarship and access to well-organized academic libraries, and relished leadership—service on the board of the National Library of Medicine on the campus of the National Institutes of Health in Bethesda, Maryland, was well worth the time and effort, and he invested a great deal of both.

Davison was serving as a consultant to the library in 1956 when the Armed Forces Medical Library, as it was then known, was renamed the National Library of Medicine and transferred to the Public Health Service.[28] The change required that the library move from its aging building on the Washington Mall to the National Institutes of Health, a campus first established in Bethesda in 1938.[29] Perhaps the move to new quarters was overdue. The library had the dubious distinction of being located in the only federal building in Washington with an outhouse[30]—until the 1887 structure was razed (not without protest)[31] and replaced by the Smithsonian's Hirshhorn Museum and Sculpture Garden, which formally opened in October 1974.[32]

Davison, pleased with his protégé's presidential appointment, offered his own jovial historical perspective. On September 25, 1970, he wrote:

> Needless to say, I was delighted that you have been appointed by Mr. Nixon as a member of the Board of Regents of the National Library of Medicine. Not only is it a very distinguished Board, but it is actually getting things accomplished through the Public Health Service which those of us who were on the previous Board could not get done through the Army. I hated to vote to turn the Surgeon General's Library over to the Public Health Service, but as a famous bank robber stated when he was asked why he robbed banks, 'You go where the money is.'[33]

Attending the annual meetings of the National Library of Medicine Board required time and travel, and McGovern's schedule in the early 1970s was already busy; but as Davison had predicted, McGovern found the library a place where important work could be accomplished. This was in large part thanks to the leadership of Martin Cummings.

Cummings, like McGovern a Duke-trained physician, was appointed director of the National Library of Medicine in the fall of 1963. This was one of John F. Kennedy's last appointments before his fateful trip to Dallas on November 22.[34] For two decades Cummings would prove a forceful leader who worked with board members like McGovern to profoundly influence the direction of medical libraries nationwide. The National Network of Libraries of Medicine that today connects nearly six thousand libraries throughout the United States was created on his watch.

In 1974, the third year of his four-year appointment, McGovern was named chairman of the board of regents, which gave him oversight of the program's then $29.7 million budget and 446 employees.[35] During his years on the board McGovern saw the flowering of such programs as MEDLINE, the national Toxicology Information Program, and the Lister Hill National Center for Biomedical Communications.[36] The Medical Library Assistance Act in particular grew under McGovern's leadership and enabled the National Library of Medicine to become a granting program providing financial support to thousands of institutions in need of library resources, staff training, research, and publications.

McGovern and his board understood that Cummings was a director who had bold ideas for the future of the library and was anxious to move it into many new areas, including the digital world that loomed on the horizon and would forever change the image of libraries from depositories of books to systems of networked electronic information.

When the "fair use" issue about photocopying for scholarly purposes was raised by large publishing houses, it was Cummings and his regents who defended the rights of health professionals employed by nonprofit institutions to photocopy journal articles for scholarly purposes.[37] A seven-year court battle carried the case to the United States Court of Claims for a 1975 ruling in favor of the National Library of Medicine and all medical libraries throughout the country.[38]

By his retirement in 1984, Cummings and his regents through the years had accomplished much. McGovern would always be proud of having followed in Davison's footsteps to make a difference for biomedical libraries and scholarship worldwide—he was, after all, like Osler and Davison a bibliophile. He collected medical books with the same joy that he had first discovered in collecting stamps as a boy. That Davison had served as a consultant guiding the National Library of Medicine's move to the National Institutes of Health and that Osler himself had been a fan and follower of the library's founder, John Shaw Billings (1838–1913), made service on the board even more meaningful to McGovern.

Billings first came to McGovern's attention through a letter Martin Cummings had sent, dated November 15, 1967.[39] Eight months earlier Cummings had been invited to Duke by Davison to present a talk titled "Books, Computers, and Three Wise Men of Medicine." Said Cummings in his cover letter to McGovern: "As requested, I am enclosing a copy of the talk I gave at Duke in which I discuss Davison's relationship with Osler." From the first line of the presentation, McGovern was hooked. It began, "Today I plan to trace the interrelationships of three eminent physicians whose common interests in books, libraries, and mechanization influenced a century of American medicine. They are Sir William Osler, the first Professor of Medicine at Johns Hopkins, Dr. John Shaw Billings, the first Director of the National Library of Medicine, and Dr. Wilburt C. Davison, the first Dean at Duke University School of Medicine."

McGovern's dog-eared and highlighted copy of that presentation speaks to his impression of Billings. That Billings directly connected with two of McGovern's lifelong heroes made him all the more a person of interest whom McGovern would talk about for years—earning him a place in this story.

To understand McGovern's love of the National Library of Medicine, one needs to go back to the end of the Civil War, when Billings, a talented

Union military surgeon who had seen service on the battlefields of Chancellorsville and Gettysburg, was transferred to Washington to assist the Office of the Surgeon General.

If you could build a city composed of only Type A personalities, John Shaw Billings would likely be elected mayor. Born in Allensville, Indiana, he was a gifted student who graduated from Miami University in 1857 at the age of fourteen and completed a medical degree from the Medical College of Ohio in 1860. What Billings accomplished in his lifetime requires an entire book to chronicle, and more than a few have been written.[40] Assigned to the army surgeon general's office in Washington, DC, in 1865, he assumed a variety of tasks for Surgeon General Joseph K. Barns (1817–1883), including inventorying post-war equipment and arms (both Union and Confederate), addressing the needs of physicians out West (including surveying their input regarding sanitation and improved fort design), organizing the Army Medical Museum, and, in his spare time, organizing and growing the surgeon general's 1,365 medical books into a functional library.[41]

Of all Billings's accomplishments, perhaps it was his organizing books into libraries and libraries into systems of libraries that earned him his widest renown and McGovern's deepest admiration. With innovative foresight and around-the-clock dedication, Billings and his staff in 1879 and 1880 organized and published *Index Medicus* (the forerunner of MEDLINE and PubMed) and the *Index Catalog,* today known as Index Cat, which provides researchers access to more than 4.5 million online medical references.[42]

William Welch, Osler's colleague and a respected dean at Hopkins, minced no words in summarizing Billings's accomplishment as "America's greatest contribution to medical knowledge."[43]

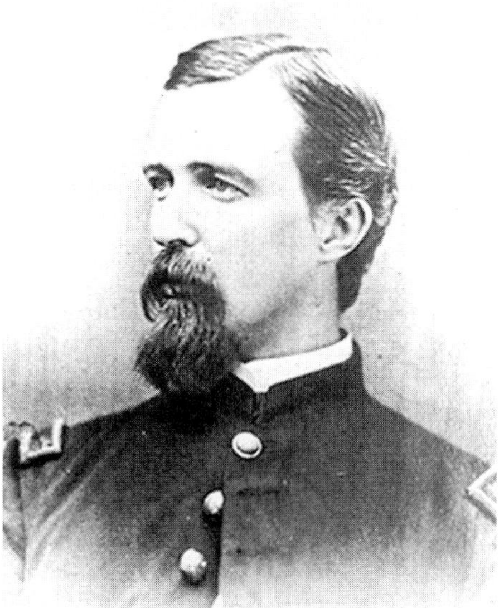

FIGURE 6.4. John Shaw Billings (1838–1913), who built the National Library of Medicine.

Sir William Osler, a close friend and admirer of Billings, watched with interest as the small library of the army surgeon general grew steadily into one of the world's great repositories of medical literature. And together Osler and Billings were instrumental in the development of other medical libraries around the world.[44] The library's reading room on Washington's Mall was a frequent stop for Osler, who had been known to lose more than a few books while riding the trains between Washington, Philadelphia, and Baltimore. On February 18, 1890, having lost a book in transit, he wrote Billings, "Bring a club with you on your next visit and pummel me well. What an aggravating devil I am? Yes, do order the book and make me pay double for it if possible."[45]

In 1974 McGovern, as chairman of the library's board of regents, would work closely with its director, Martin Cummings, to lead the library Billings had built into the digital age. Billings had labored through the nights penciling stacks of journal articles and books with his instructions for indexing their content. Now McGovern was putting Billings's work to use in a new technological age as computers revolutionized every aspect of medical libraries, from indexing to acquisition of content.

Today medical professionals around the world access the National Library of Medicine's collections using sophisticated computer programs known as PubMed and MEDLARS,[46] which are direct descendents of Billings's early hand-indexed catalogs. Billings and Osler alike would marvel at the instant access to medical literature available on the desktop now at the click of a mouse. Cummings, McGovern, and the library's regents readily adopted every technological advantage in the evolution of information management.

While much of his attention in the early 1970s was focused on service to the National Library of Medicine, closer to home McGovern also set his sights on improving the Houston Academy of Medicine–Texas Medical Center Library (HAM–TMC), which is today one of eight regional libraries of the National Library of Medicine and is one of the largest medical libraries in the world.[47]

In 1969—the same year President Nixon requested McGovern's service at the National Library of Medicine—McGovern was named curator of rare books at the HAM–TMC Library. Today the John P. McGovern Rare Book Collection in the Texas Medical Center contains over 18,500 volumes, including direct gifts from McGovern's personal collection and from other donors, in addition to books obtained through his funding support.[48] This collection focuses primarily on the development of the medical specialties in the late nineteenth and early twentieth centuries and includes McGovern's collection of more than a thousand Osler-related books, along with a fireplace mantel recovered from the basement of Osler's Oxford home at 13 Norham Gardens.

Elizabeth White, now retired, was the founding director of rare books and archives for the HAM–TMC Library. She remembers how well McGovern was acquainted with his books long after he had donated them to the rare books collection that bears his name. "He read and knew them," she said. "Many times he would call me at the library and say, 'I'm looking for this quote. I know it's in such-and-such a book, probably about the second or third chapter.'" White would go off to find the quote, and whether at "the end of the third chapter or the beginning of the fourth chapter . . . that quote would be just about right where he said it was. He not only collected, he knew his books."[49]

Doctor of Giving

On January 1, 1986, Jack McGovern retired from his clinical practice, which he sold to his senior associates, including Ted Haywood, the best man at his wedding. Later his associates relocated the practice in leased facilities a few miles farther west of the Medical Center, but they continue to prosper within eyeshot of it, under the name McGovern Allergy and Asthma Clinic. In the front lobby of the clinic a large portrait of McGovern greets every patient.

In time McGovern sold the land and clinic building he had occupied near the Medical Center to the Kelsey-Seybold Clinic, that large, multispecialty enterprise founded by Mavis Kelsey, who had once provided the clinic space McGovern needed as Kelsey moved to larger quarters. Now it was McGovern's turn to provide the ever-expanding Kelsey-Seybold Clinic (today a network of twenty clinics and nearly four hundred physicians[50]) the land it needed to build a new $70 million clinical complex near the Texas Medical Center.[51]

John McGovern had accomplished much during his professional life. As son, physician, medical educator, Oslerian, historian, writer and editor, researcher, businessman, rare medical-book collector, early contributor to the growth and reputation of the Texas Medical Center, citizen giving of his time and his foundation's money to innumerable community causes, and devoted husband, McGovern had come a long way from his early days in Washington, DC, playing for marbles.

As he had planned all along, in retirement he now had the resources of his foundation (which was valued at more than $180 million at the time of his death in 2007) with which to switch roles from doctor of patients to doctor of giving. For the nineteen years that he lived after retiring, he would keep Orville Story and the foundation staff busy as the foundation continued to make money and to bestow it on the medical community and the community at large.

After McGovern retired, he and Kathy would spend part of the year in their beloved home in Indian Wells, California, adjacent to Palm Springs, where they built many strong and lasting friendships. The rest of the time they spent in Houston, where they lived a quiet and private life shared with close friends they had known through the years.

McGovern suffered a near-fatal heart attack in Houston in 1996. It was clear that he might well have died had he been traveling at the time. Being in Houston, close to his personal physicians and within minutes of the critical-care capabilities of the Texas Medical Center, probably saved his life. Once during the weeklong ordeal his heart actually stopped beating, requiring emergency action by the medical team to revive him.

Following his close brush with death, the resilient McGovern bounced back with a renewed appreciation of life (and a carefully controlled diet) that translated into working even harder for his foundation, a passion for which kept him busy day and night through the remaining decade of his life. Slowing him down proved nearly impossible for those around him, although they constantly tried. In 1999 the McGoverns would sell their home in California, but they kept their high-rise condominium next to the Texas Medical Center, along with their latest home on Galveston Island, which they had bought in 1998.[52]

McGovern spent his last decade close to the beach and in the salt air he and Kathy had always loved, where walks along the water and memories of great fish caught or lost always gave him pleasure. And always there was the foundation and the joy of making the right investment at the right time for some gain that would provide funds to support good causes.

And McGovern never ran out of good causes.

Consider the fact that on any given day, hundreds of school children (more than thirty thousand annually[53]) are visiting the John P. McGovern

Museum of Health & Medical Science in Houston's Museum District to learn about the human body and the value of preventive medicine; one of eleven faculty holding an endowed McGovern professorship is teaching the next generation of health professionals; and a family is visiting the Houston Zoo where they stop by the McGovern Lake and the McGovern Children's Zoo and perhaps catch a glimpse of a Masai giraffe born at the zoo and named "Jack" in McGovern's honor. In Washington a Nobel Laureate or Supreme Court Justice who is a member of the Cosmos Club may be using the McGovern Library or attending a McGovern endowed lecture. At Duke University students are trotting in and out of buildings on the medical campus bearing the name "McGovern-Davison"—all made possible from McGovern Foundation funds.

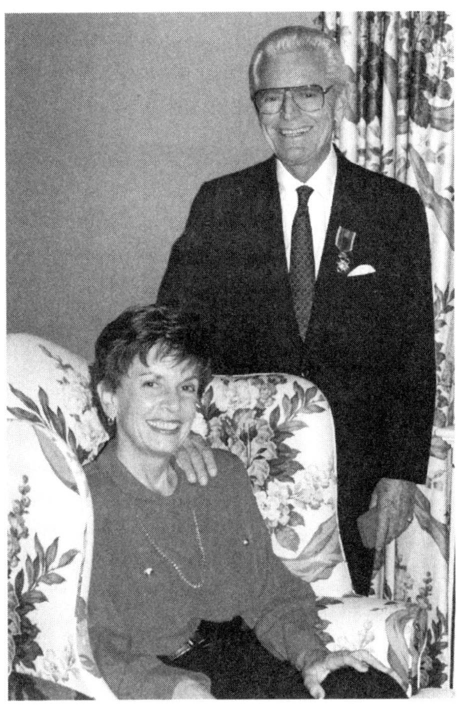

FIGURE 6.5. John P. McGovern and wife, Kathy McGovern, 1988.

In England, Osler's famous home at 13 Norham Gardens, Oxford, has been renovated to include the Osler-McGovern Centre and returned to use as a gathering place for scholarly workshops. Scholars from universities worldwide gather in the home where Osler once shared his books and love of medicine with students like Wilburt Davison. Conferences gather at Green Templeton College in memory of Osler's "latch-key" philosophy. McGovern's foundation has helped make all this possible.

In the Texas Medical Center students and faculty from all institutions and disciplines can be found dining together in the McGovern Commons. The leaders of the Texas Medical Center conduct meetings with international visitors on the McGovern Campus, once the home to a Nabisco bakery that the foundation retooled and modernized into office space for Texas Medical Center institutions.

Students at the University of Texas Health Science Center at Houston, with its six professional schools, are enriching their education through the McGovern Center for Humanities and Ethics. Students at the Institute for Medical Humanities at the UT Medical Branch in Galveston are attending lectures on the history of medicine or participating in innovative medical humanities and ethics programs endowed by McGovern in the spirit of the art and the science of health-care delivery.

Out in the community, a family hoping to foster a child in need is meeting with a social worker whose salary is supported by a gift from McGovern's foundation. There is a reading circle for children over at the McGovern/Stella Link Library, a Houston public library near the Medical Center named in McGovern's honor. McGovern teaching awards, McGovern student awards, McGovern lectures—the list of awards, honors, professorships, and facilities named for McGovern is as long as it is diverse and requires an appendix to this book to present (appendix C).

Perhaps the physician from DC who preferred not to be called a philanthropist might find "doctor of giving" more acceptable. After all, the gift of giving was one of his greatest legacies.

Chapter Seven

Last Glimpses

No human being is constituted to know the truth, the whole truth, and nothing but the truth; and even the best of men must be content with fragments, with partial glimpses, never the full fruition. —WILLIAM OSLER, 1905[1]

Up Close and Personal

The stories of John McGovern's life tell us much about the man, but do they answer the question whether we really know him or know only what we want to know?

Even the great Osler was no saint. From time to time he was criticized by the media, even battered in the popular press.[2] William Bean, a lifelong Oslerian and the first president of the American Osler Society, insisted, "To me Osler was no paper saint, but a very human person. His imp of the perverse sustained a streak of practical joking which made many people miserable and got him into a world of trouble."[3]

Osler freely admitted, "I have made mistakes, but they have been mistakes of the head not of the heart."[4] McGovern, like Osler, was certainly no stranger to his own mistakes, as he demonstrated amply during his parents' Thanksgiving visit to Durham, when he rewarded their time, trouble, and long anticipation by disappearing into his lab and abandoning them to his roommate. And we saw a temperamental side to McGovern as a young faculty member who engaged in an "altercation" in a parking lot. Nor was that the only occasion on which his temper got the best of him.

McGovern was as complex as he was talented. Those who worked with him daily are quick to praise his fairness and his work ethic but are mindful that he was the Chief—with a capital "C"—who called the shots. From early on he was recognized as driven,[5] and his drive only intensified in the course of his career. As a physician he was gentle and compassionate. As a businessman investing money and building his foundation, he was often forceful and demanding. That he could balance medical and business careers simultaneously and be extraordinarily successful at both is impressive, to say the least.

Orville Story, who spent so many years providing the numbers that guided McGovern's business decisions, knew McGovern the businessman better than anybody else did, and he had great admiration for his boss. Yet Story was quick to note that the two had their battles from time to time. On one occasion, "Mrs. McGovern had to come downstairs to serve as referee to break up our shouting match by reminding us both how many years we had worked together so productively and that a good night's rest would do us both a great deal of good. She was right. The next day we couldn't remember what got us both so agitated with each other."[6] The tireless and sometimes mercurial McGovern could test the patience and endurance of even the most loyal of employees.

Glenn Knotts (1935–2003), a distinguished Purdue alum[7] and close friend of McGovern's, who assisted with foundation projects for several years, recalled that the Chief could dish out his displeasure in generous portions, and he was particularly quick to do so if he suspected an employee of presenting him with sloppy research. In fact any evidence of slipshod performance could bring down a rain of fire. "We got into such a shouting match one afternoon in Galveston that I announced my resignation, slammed the door, and drove to the nearest beach, where I paced back and forth until the sun went down."

The next week, recalled Knotts, "We had lunch together and the matter was dropped, never to surface again."[8]

On a sunny July afternoon in 1996, Knotts was shot three times as his car was hijacked at a carwash near the Texas Medical Center on the corner of Kirby Drive and North Braeswood.[9] The unknown assailant dragged

Knotts out of the driver's seat and sped away in his car, leaving Knotts to crawl to the now locked door of the adjacent gas station while onlookers gasped in horror. "I just sat on the curb in a pool of blood and waited to die," he recalled. He had a vague recollection of paramedics and demanding to be taken to Hermann Hospital, where trauma surgeon Red Duke found that one of the bullets had missed his spinal column by millimeters.[10] Knotts survived.

Years later, with tears standing in his eyes, Knotts relived that close encounter with death. In the aftermath of the most terrible experience of his life, Knotts found that the person among his friends who emerged as the warmest and the most caring was Jack McGovern. Said Knotts, who would die from colon cancer just six years later,[11] "He could at times be impossible to work with, but always, without question, he was loyal to his friends and colleagues."[12]

Few employees over the years were closer to McGovern than Julia Mitchell, who joined his clinic in August 1973 as a staff nurse. By January 1976 she was working afternoons in McGovern's office on the second floor of the clinic and had been permanently moved into the role of administrative assistant:

> I went up temporarily in the afternoons to help him answer phones because his long-time secretary, Norma Stone, had left. That was just supposed to be temporary. . . . Dr. McGovern was a very unique person to work for. You made no independent decisions, everything was through him, and some people can't work like that. I tried to stay half a step behind him. You could never stay in front of him, but you tried to—and you had to have everything just in line. He used to have stacks of correspondence on his desk. I could tell you what was in each stack because when he wanted something, you had to know where it was. . . . You had to keep records, you had to be accurate, you had to stay on top of things, and you had to notice things that needed to be done.[13]

Mitchell not only stayed on top of things, she became an indispensable organizer of McGovern's busy clinical and business agenda, juggling complex travel schedules and day-to-day details with the precision he expected. To manage all the irons he plunged simultaneously into the fire,

McGovern "really kept to the Osler system of living in 'day-tight compartments,'" Mitchell says:

> He always talked to me about that. He would be doing patients, he would be doing the oversight of the entire clinic, and he would be doing publications, serving on many, many boards and committees. Doctor [as Mitchell and the other office staff referred to McGovern throughout their working relationship and after his death] never really took vacation. He would say vacation, but vacation for him meant working fifty to fifty-five hours a week instead of working the normal seventy or eighty. . . . he was an early riser, and he did not stop. He always had multiple, multiple, multiple things going on.[14]

Despite his obsessive work habits that often kept his staff busy into the small hours, McGovern was also known to be surprisingly thoughtful about the needs of his staff's family and children. When her son Kevin was born, Mitchell was prepared to give up her job. McGovern quickly found ways to keep her on, even when it meant bringing the child to work, where he played and napped in the kitchen attached to McGovern's office.

Four decades later, Mitchell remains on the foundation board assisting Kathy McGovern with the legacy of giving that McGovern began.

Gail Glass, who went to work for McGovern in 1975 and stayed for more than three decades, says this:

> I was doing a lot of his typing and his speeches. I did secretarial work, whatever was needed for the clinic part, along with any letters or anything that he needed typed. . . . We normally did about nine rewrites of anything he did. That was pretty much par for the course. And he did a lot of speeches at that time, too, when I first came . . . but you couldn't use the correction tape on a carbon, and lots of letters we did for the clinic were an original and four copies, because we had no Xerox machine in those days.
>
> He was always kind to me. I have nothing but good memories of working for him. At Christmas we had what we called a 'gathering,' where the entire staff would go down to the lobby on Brompton. Kathy had wrapped a gift for everyone, and you received your Christmas bonus. But when he gave you your gift or your bonus, he knew something individually about

everybody, and there were about 110 of us at that point. It was amazing that he knew everyone personally, or knew something about them to comment on. That always impressed me.[15]

When Glass found herself unexpectedly raising an additional child in her growing family, McGovern stepped in and helped with some hospital costs and child care, an act of kindness that she could never talk about, given a firm McGovern rule that office talk about compensation and money matters was grounds for dismissal.[16]

Bill McLemore, supervisor of McGovern's clinic laboratory, started working for McGovern back in 1958 at the original clinic on Montrose in a small broom closet converted into a working lab. He stayed on for the next fifty years, retiring (to part-time status) in December 2010. McLemore remembers that in 1965, when the clinic moved from Montrose to Travis Street, closer to the Medical Center, McGovern gave him one of the eleven coveted covered parking places, with the agreement that physicians joining the practice would move him down the line until the last covered spot was taken. Each time a new physician joined the practice, McLemore moved his car down the line, until he arrived at the last covered parking spot. But his expectation of losing the spot was never fulfilled, as the large Brompton clinic opened, and everyone moved to new parking and office space.[17]

While McGovern was frugal and signed every check in the early days of the clinic, with final approval on every purchase down to the office chairs, McLemore recalls one incident involving McGovern and money that surprised him.

We had a meeting one day while the clinic was still on Travis with the head bookkeeper at the time, Ray Bookwalter. He was telling us that anything we needed we could have, but don't order anything that we didn't direly need. He was trying to keep the expenses down as much as we could. So I went to Ray and told him if he needed to, he could cut my salary. I would be glad to do that. And Ray said, 'Well, let me tell him.' So he told Dr. McGovern and McGovern said, 'No that's not what I wanted to do. I'm going to give Bill a one-hundred-dollar raise for offering to do that.' So he gave me a hundred-dollar-a-month raise for offering to take a salary cut.[18]

Gay Collette (1945–2011), a native of Alvin, Texas, and a loyal employee of McGovern's for more than thirty-five years, went to work for him at the new Brompton clinic.

> When I started, there were these trays of the old ledger accounts, and I started looking through them, and I thought, Oh, my goodness, how on earth am I going to even start, because they were so old. . . . Dr. McGovern had never pursued any means of collecting this money. They would send letters with statements, but he never pushed. So it was a very delicate balancing act to set up some type of collection procedure to bring some of this money in, and, of course, I had to have everything approved by him because, again, he did not want to just start off with hard collections. So we set up different messages on the statements, and then I would start calling some of the patients and just find out if there was a problem that was not reflected on the ledger sheets. So that's how it started.[19]

Within a few years, in the mid-1980s, Collette had a computer that would instantly make her life easier. Or so she thought.

> I'll never forget the first statements that went out on our computers. I don't know what happened, but everybody got a delinquent message, even our current and good patients. And, oh, the phones were ringing off the wall. So we started looking back, and, yes, somehow in the computer program there was a glitch, and all we could do was apologize.
>
> So of course we had to bring Doctor in and explain what had happened. We expected him just to explode. He did not. He came in there and he said, "Okay. How can we salvage the situation?" And he never got upset. He just thought through the process, he understood what had happened, that it was not our fault, that it was the case that the programmers had just not put in some little data information that was needed. . . . So now our goal was to salvage, and so we just sent a letter to everybody explaining that this was our first run from our new computers, and we apologized for any unnecessary grief and that the message that they got . . . was not meant to be that way, but through error it happened. So we salvaged.[20]

"Salvage" is a word used by more than a few of McGovern's longtime employees. When day-to-day problems arose in the business of running the clinic, employees knew that McGovern would search for a solution rather than a culprit, and that he would find it fast. In this way he built a reputation for fairness, and a stock of loyalty among his employees.

Up close and personally, Jack McGovern was all business and in a constant state of movement, spurred by an insatiable work ethic that did not distinguish day from night. He never knew a slack tide when it came to work, and what was a full day of work for many was a half day to him. He liked diligence and disliked wasting time. His staff knew that his dislikes included meetings (unless he called them), and more than a few times he had been known to ask employees chatting in the hall or at the coffee pot, "Who called this meeting?" It was his mild reminder that there are only so many hours in a day, and he called the meetings.

"The master-word is Work, a little one, as I have said," Osler asserted in his famous essay "Aequanimitas," "but fraught with momentous consequences if you can but write it on the tablets of your hearts, and bind it upon your foreheads."[21] McGovern, Julia Mitchell recalls, modeled that master word around the clock. Good medical care was not acceptable; it had to be better than good, and work was what made it so. "Even the design of the Brompton clinic was such that patients could see the medical staff was busy and serving others while they waited. If a patient asked a question, you never [said] 'I don't know,' and just let it go. You always said, 'I don't know, but I'll be glad to find out. I'll be right back.'"[22]

McGovern's clinical care, teaching, research, and academic work around the country were conducted in the public eye. But his business side—the side that invested and that built the foundation—was one few saw. Weekends and holidays provided time for reviewing his investment strategies for the coming week. Having no children of his own and focused as he was, he often imperfectly separated his work schedule from the downtime of others, even on Christmas. He was known to call stock brokers assigned to him by major Wall Street firms on Christmas morning and Easter, since the stock market exchange was closed then and it was a good time to discuss and give directives. Playing for all the marbles was more than a childhood pass time—it was a major theme of his life.

Gay Collette, who had successfully dealt with the computer billing glitches of the mid-1980s, moved to the foundation side of the business by the early 1990s and knew McGovern's tireless approach to investments as well as anyone. "When he committed to buying something," she says, "he was going to do it on his terms, and he did. He would put all of his energy in it. I know Mr. Story would be on the phone, they'd hang up, he'd call back, they'd hang up, call back—it was ongoing until it was a done deal. And then he would just move on to the next topic."[23]

Sometimes McGovern needed some pushback from the staff, and only those who had worked close to him for years would dare to supply it. Gay Collette was one who dared.

> Gosh, I dreaded those days so bad, days when he would want to work relentlessly into the night. Finally, one day we had just been at it and at it and at it, and he was getting a little testy and I was getting testy in return, and I told him, I said, "Doctor, I've had enough for today. I can't do this anymore, so I'm going home." And the next day when he called he said, "How are you today?" I said, "I'm fine. I'm much better, thank you." And he would just laugh. Doctor didn't apologize very often, but when he knew he overstepped his boundaries—and that was one time—he said, "I'm sorry."
>
> He always worked. I think from the minute he opened his eyes until he went to bed, seven days a week, he would work. And his mind was always working. . . . before he purchased a piece of property, Doctor tore it apart and put it together—numbers—just always working with numbers and pushing the last button to get what he wanted out of the transaction. . . . He was born with that sense, and he would read *Forbes* magazine, he would read the *Wall Street Journal,* and he would listen to the *Business Hour* on PBS. Those were his favorite media communications.[24]

Taking calls from McGovern on Christmas morning did not fit the lifestyle of a number of the brokers assigned by large investment firms to coordinate his weekly directives. Gay Collette knew that well: "He had to go through a couple of brokers to get the right one that could work with him, and that would be Jeanette Mattiza. . . . She was the first female that worked with him. She had known of his buying and selling when she was in [her firm's] cash management office, and then once she became a broker she worked just for him, nobody else."[25]

Jeanette Mattiza remembers the transition in 1993 when her investment firm gave her the assignment to work with McGovern:

> I was a little shell-shocked, should I say. I was coming out of a comfort zone. . . . But he was very warm and welcoming. He always was very inquisitive about family and very personable that way, so even though you thought you were meeting with someone that was several levels above you, he had a way of making you feel comfortable. . . .
>
> Everything he did, I think, connected back to his scientist's thinking, so working with him you would realize where he was coming from, because he would analyze everything, just as he did with his research. If it was repeatable, could be proven, everything was fine. But if it didn't make sense, it's not going to happen. . . . So it was always digging deeper to get to the bottom of why and how it worked, and then he would make a decision based on all of that. But I think it was just because of his scientist's mind.
>
> . . . I don't know where he found the time to do it. He must have just been thinking all the time. . . . If you can imagine, detailed buy-and-sell prices on various things in the little black book. His handwriting was very, very neat, and these books were not very big. That's how he kept a record of all the facts.[26]

Language was important to McGovern. He fussed over every word while his staff typed as many as nine drafts of a document late into the night, and he was equally careful about numbers. He had the gift of never forgetting a number—especially when currency was involved. Words and numbers were both tools with special meanings and had to be used accordingly. In his world of investments, no number should change without explanation; to give McGovern a number and change it without explanation was unacceptable.

Business was business, and McGovern could be tough—even downright unpleasant—when either numbers or the terms of an agreement did not line up. Some investments involved partnerships on big building projects in and outside of Texas. It simply didn't matter how far back a working relationship with someone went or how deep the trust ran—if one piece of a deal was out of place, McGovern moved quickly and minced no words. He lost patience with one individual, for instance, when what he saw as thumb-twiddling on this man's part and imperfect fidelity to an initial agreement between them formed a combustible mixture. The result was a controlled explosion. "For well over a year," he wrote Waughtal,

> I have had numerous discussions with you and my tax and legal advisors concerning the problems surrounding the two captioned limited partnerships.
>
> . . . The professional demands upon my time are great, in terms of my physical, emotional, and intellectual reserves. . . . These matters have significantly added to my burdens, jeopardized and adversely affected my tax planning and have caused my bookkeeper, my tax consultant, my attorney, as well as myself, great additional expenditures in time, effort and in money.
>
> In spite of every inclination to the contrary, I am forced to say that the offer which I made by telephone to you concerning [these properties], is hereby revoked, and that any further discussions or questions concerning these deals must be referred to my attorney."[27]

He then signed the letter, "As always, with best personal regards."

McGovern could be as forceful and focused as he could be charming and personable. It was a skill set required of a person working in what would appear to be the immiscible worlds of clinical care and high-stakes investing. Those who worked close to McGovern's core and knew his moods could find themselves simultaneously frustrated and mesmerized. His sense of humor, too, depended on what he was doing. When he was conducting investment business, it could be hard to find. Recalls Orville Story:

> Well, he did have a sense of humor, but it was mostly dealing with people that had nothing to do with his business. He was so sincere and serious about what was going on, there was very little opportunity to have light talk. I know, for example, he and I would eat dinner and I would direct the conversation to something about baseball, football, basketball, or some issue that would be light enough that we could get away from the heavy. I would trap him into talking about that a little bit, but all of a sudden it would hit him, 'Hey, we're wasting time, here—let's get back to business.' But he did have a sense of humor, and he kept up with a lot of the sports.[28]

While McGovern played for all the marbles, it should be noted that he did not win every agate he had set his eye on when it came to real estate investments. Story recalled McGovern's exasperation when he met his match on one real estate deal in the early 1960s, just down the street from the Texas Medical Center near the Houston landmark of the day, the Shamrock Hilton Hotel. He had been buying houses in the area with the intention of one day owning a large enough block of property to accommodate his own clinic building in coming years. But to his chagrin, an elderly widow who owned the last piece of property he needed also knew how to play for all the marbles. Story chortled as he recalled the sale that never happened:

> Her father had always told her it would be worth X number of dollars, which was outlandish. We ended up selling the whole Block 5, except for that one site, and the developer that bought that also went to work on this lady . . . and they never got it. . . . We kept telling her what it was going to be like if she didn't sell—the term was "the bowels" of the development—which means where the garbage trucks would come in and out and all that. That didn't faze her. She just kept it, and I guess her heirs still have it.[29]

While McGovern was frustrated by the outcome of the negotiations, no doubt he grudgingly admired the widow for holding her ground and keeping her agate. Shortly after this misadventure, on a trip to Miami, he received a call from his friend Jack Trotter and learned that another tract of property nearby was available, owned by Jim West. Trotter proposed that it could be bought and split among investors if McGovern wanted in.[30]

McGovern quickly took ownership of the prize section of the property and held his share—the future home of his new allergy clinic at the corner of Holcombe Boulevard and Brompton.

Looking back on McGovern's life, one wonders how he evaluated it himself when he neared its end. The best answer may come from Billy F. Andrews. Chairman emeritus of pediatrics at the University of Louisville School of Medicine, Andrews had trained with Davison and had known McGovern since medical school. He made a visit to Houston in 2005, just two years before McGovern died. Late into the night he and McGovern relived favorite stories about Davison, Duke medical school days, and Sir William Osler. The talk grew deep and reflective. McGovern rose from his chair to retire for the night, then paused and spoke some parting words. Andrews later put them to paper as best he could remember them and framed them for his office wall.

"We have been most fortunate in our lives," McGovern said, "to have such wonderful careers, great mentors, beautiful and wonderful wives, good friends, and challenges and opportunities to fulfill.

"To serve and to love are the greatest action and ethical verbs in our language. And to serve and to love are the greatest ideals for medicine and life."[31]

In that remark McGovern touched on the main lights in his life: his career, which included both medicine and the business that enabled his philanthropy; Davison; Kathy; friends; and challenges—hills to climb. He had loved and he had served. Looking back over his life, he had the satisfaction of knowing that he had lived it well.

Full Circle

And now these stories of the life of John P. McGovern have come full circle. As I stand beside him in the cold hospital room, the only life I see is in the motion and sounds of machines that track his vital signs. It is the last day of May 2007, only two days short of his eighty-sixth birthday.

His body, old and frail, has finally given out. What first appeared as a cold is now full-blown pneumonia. The best medications failed to turn the tide during that Memorial Day weekend, and I now find myself beside him—not to share a good story, but to share a moment of silence as he slips away.

Outside, spring is quickly yielding to summer. The sky is clear and the air is growing hotter. Galveston beaches with seagulls screaming overhead are crowded with families, the children looking forward to the summer vacation before them. Inside this room, there is little to look forward to; I can only wonder if he is here at all. That high-energy, nonstop mind of his seems still, and the vacuum he has left seems to be sucking the air right out of the room. It is that dreaded moment we must all face, and he is in the moment.

At times like this, one thinks of the strangest things. Kathy is sitting tearful across the room from him. Julia Mitchell and Gay Collette are out in the hall pacing silently. And I am standing over him thinking of beach-house and Glenn Knotts stories. It seems strange that I am not with the others in the hall, but in here with him thinking of stories. But I cannot convince myself that he is entirely gone.

My mind flashes back to a day just a year earlier, but a lifetime away. I had driven down to Galveston to visit my friend and on an impulse had taken my five-year-old daughter with me. It was a first-time visit for her, and driving down, I wondered if it was a mistake to inflict a high-energy five-year-old on a fragile, elderly man. But since the early days when, a schoolboy himself, he had followed his father on rounds and peered through the glass at the newborns at Garfield Hospital, there had been an understanding between McGovern and children. In his beachfront retreat he was deprived of their company; and so I took her.

It was not a mistake.

McGovern's face was wreathed in smiles as he watched her run headlong and carefree around the room. Without putting a limit on how many she could take, he offered her candies from a big bowl on the coffee table, and howled with laughter when her fist emerged clamped around more candy than any tiny fingers should have been able to hold. A few minutes later she was perched on his chair, and the two, the young and the old, were the image of shared delight. What a joyful moment—now a world away.

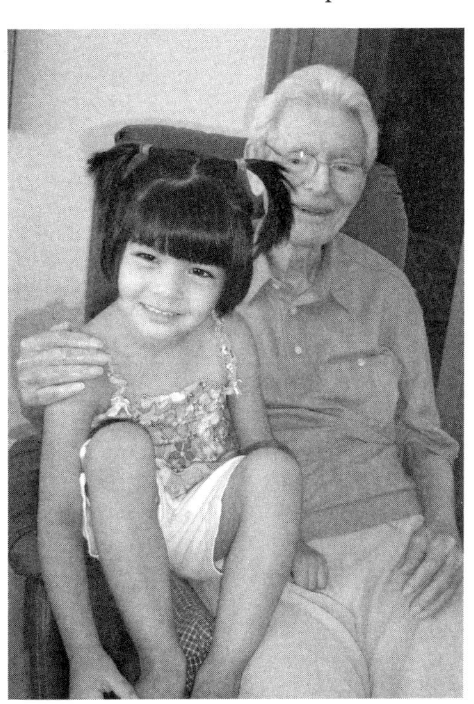

FIGURE 7.1. McGovern with newfound friend.

And looking down at him, unsure whether he is there or not, I think of another story, one from two decades earlier. Lee Clark—who as a young man had awakened on the grounds of Emory University to the sight of a glowing pink monument in the sunrise, and had built his great hospital with that image in his mind—had suffered a stroke and in the first few months could not communicate, but lay tightly locked in his unresponsive body. He would survive the stroke by six years, and with the help of therapists would regain partial use of his voice and some mobility. But McGovern had been deeply troubled when he first learned of Clark's condition, of that brilliant mind, working around the clock, yet unable to communicate a single word.

Shortly after Clark's stroke, McGovern was at his weekly lunch meeting with Glenn Knotts, who told me the story. McGovern sat in the busy Chinese restaurant at midday, ignoring his food, and wanting to talk only about Clark's situation. He could not shake it off. To be "trapped in your own body," unable to communicate, however minutely, was a fate terrible beyond imagining. Working himself into a state of great distress, and oblivious to the staring diners around him, he bellowed, "Glenn, if that happened to me, would you just get a gun and shoot me? I would shoot you!"

Then, suddenly becoming conscious of the dismay he had created with his outburst—alarmed diners were pausing with forks midair—he grinned and let it go.

Yet here he was on this, his last day, hooked to an interminable array of monitors and tubes. The man with unbounded energy and an endless torrent of ideas was silent. But was he still there, with all his mental faculties, unable to speak as he had feared he one day would be? Or was he somewhere else, looking joyfully across a shrinking divide at Granny Brown, Mac and Lottie, Helen, Dean Davison—ringed in light?

Just before noon, McGovern died.[32]

HIS PORTRAIT HANGS on the wall overlooking my keyboard as I tell these stories about his life. There is a slight grin on his face, his eyes make contact. The speckled trout I once gave him to hang in his study now swims again across my own. Jack McGovern was my mentor and my friend. He was a collector and a doer—and a man who played for all the marbles. He won most of them.

And then, as carefully as he had won them, he gave them away.

Appendix A

Awards and Honors

ACADEMIC HONORS

Phi Beta Kappa
Alpha Omega Alpha
Sigma Pi Sigma

HONORARY DEGREES

Ricker College, ScD, 1971
Union College, LLD, 1972
Kent State University, LHD, 1973
University of Nebraska, ScD, 1973
Illinois College of Podiatric Medicine, DPM, 1975
Lincoln College, LittD, 1976
Emerson College, LHD, 1976
Ball State University, ScD, 1977
Huston-Tillotson College, ScD, 1977
John F. Kennedy University, DPhil, 1978
Limestone College, DMedSc, 1979
Southeastern University, DPhil, 1979
Texas Christian University, DHS, 1981
Georgetown University, ScD, 1981
William Penn College, DHumMed, 1982

Catawba College, DHS, 1983
Florida State University, ScD, 1984
Lamar University, LLD, 1984
Alaska Pacific University, DPS, 1985
Houston Graduate School of Theology, LHD, 1986
Troy State University, LLD, 1986
Pan American University, LLD, 1987
Thomas Jefferson University, Jefferson Medical College, LittD, 1987
University of the City of Manila, ScD, 1989
National University of Cordoba (Argentina), DMed, 1990
Florida A&M University, SD, 1991
Southern Vermont College, LLD, 1991
Centenary College, LHD, 1995
Duke University, ScD, 1995

PROFESSIONAL HONORS

The Borden Undergraduate Research Award in Medicine, Duke University School of Medicine ("for meritorious research completed during his medical training"), 1945

Sigma Xi, The Scientific Research Society of America, 1948
- Chairman, Zone 7 Committee (Texas, Louisiana, Arkansas, Oklahoma)
- Panel of Consultants for the Chapter-at-Large, 1967–1970
- Member, National Committee on the Membership-at-Large, 1970–1975
- Nominating Committee (National Officers), 1972–1974; Chairman, 1972
- Member, Board of Directors, 1972–1973
- Chairman, Proctor Medal Committee (RESA)

John and Mary Markle Scholar in Medical Science, 1950–1955

Smith-Reed-Russell Medical Honor Society, George Washington University School of Medicine, Honorary Member, 1951. (One faculty member elected each year by students as "Outstanding Teacher of the Year.")

Walter Reed Society, 1951–1964
- Vice President, 1952–1953

William Beaumont Medical Society, Washington, DC, Honorary Member, 1952

Governor's Appointee, White House Conference on Children and Youth, 1960

Alpha Epsilon Delta (National Honorary Pre-Medical Society), Honorary Member, 1961

Westchester Allergy Society (New York), Honorary Member, 1968

Governor's Appointee, White House Conference on Children and Youth, 1970

Bela Schick Memorial Address, Recipient Bela Schick Gold Medal Award, 1970

Enuresis Foundation Award for the "most significant research" on the subject, 1970

First Distinguished Award of Merit, American College of Allergists, for "extraordinary and meritorious contribution to the field of allergy," 27th Annual Congress, San Francisco, 1970

Eta Sigma Gamma (National Professional Health Science Society) National Honor Award, elected first National Honorary Member, October 1973

Clemens von Pirquet Award and Lecture, Georgetown University Medical Center, 1975

John P. McGovern Award for Meritorious Contributions and Service, first recipient, Texas School Health Association, 1977

Pi Kappa Alpha Fraternity, 1939–1983
- Distinguished Achievement Award, 1986
- Order of the West Range, 1994
- Sabre & Key Society, 1997

The Chauncey Leake History of Medicine Society, Honorary Member, University of Texas Medical Branch, Galveston, Texas, 1985

Thomas Linacre Medal in Medical Humanities, Joseph and Rose Kennedy Institute of Ethics, Georgetown University, 1986

Omicron Delta Kappa, Troy State University Circle, Honorary Member, 1987

Robert E. Gross Humanitarian Award of the Foundation for Children, 1988

Harold Swanberg Distinguished Service Award, American Medical Writers Association, 1988

Fred Schwengel Award, the highest award of the Historical Research Foundation of Washington, DC, 1988

Certificate of Commendation from the US Department of Health and Human Services/Public Health Services, 1988

American Medical Association Education and Research Foundation Award 1988

Spirit of Margaret Mead Award, Institute for Intercultural Studies, 1989

Outstanding Scholarship in Health Care Award, American Association of Colleges of Nursing, 1990

Association for Medical Education and Research in Substance Abuse, Honorary Member, 1991

First Recovery Movement Humanitarian Award, Desert Rehab Services, 1995

R. Brinkley Smithers Gold Medal Award, National Council on Alcoholism and Drug Dependence, 1996

Outstanding Retired Physician Award, first recipient, Retired Physician's Organization of the Harris County Medical Society, 1997

Exemplary Efforts in Drug Prevention Award, Houston's Drug-Free Business Initiative, 1997

President's Award, Council on Alcohol & Drug Abuse/Houston, 1997

Japan Osler Society, Honorary Member, 1998

NACoA Sustainer Recognition Award, National Association for Children of Alcoholics, 1999

National Leadership Award, American Society of Addiction Medicine, 2001

The Ambassador Leonard K. Firestone Award of Merit, ABC Recovery Center, Indio, California, 2002

Robin Bush Award, Bo's Place (grief counseling center for children who have lost loved ones), Houston, 2003

TEAM Spirit Award, Kick Drugs Out of America (a.k.a. KICKSTART), 2003

Excellence in Medicine President's Award, American Medical Association Foundation, 2007

PERSONAL HONORS

Smith-Reed-Russell Medical Honor Society, George Washington University School of Medicine, Honorary Member, 1951. (One faculty member elected each year by students as "Outstanding Teacher of the Year.")

Distinguished Service Award, American School Health Association, 1973

Distinguished Alumni Award, Duke University School of Medicine, 1976

Investiture Award and Address, West Virginia School of Medicine, 1977

Appreciation Reminiscences and Tributes Honoring John P. McGovern, Ovid Bell Press, 1980, 680 pages, presented to McGovern by friends, students, and colleagues on his fifty-fifth birthday

Award and Commencement Address, School of Allied Health Science, University of Texas Houston Health Science Center, 1981

Testimonial Dinner and Award (Baylor College of Medicine, University of Texas Health Science Center at Houston, University of Texas M. D. Anderson Cancer Center, and Texas Medical Center) for "more than 25 years of highly meritorious service as professor in each of our institutions," Doctor's Club, Houston, Texas, 1981

Distinguished Service Award, Coalition of National Health Education Organizations, 1982

William A. Howe Award, American School Health Association, 1983

The Private Sector Initiative Commendation from President Ronald Reagan, March 6, 1985

Medical Library Association, Honorary Member, 1985 (fourth Honorary Membership conferred by Medical Library Association since its founding in 1898)

Distinguished Alumnus Award, Alpha Epsilon Delta (National Premedical Honor Society), 1986

Lamp of Learning Award, University of Texas at Austin School of Nursing, 1987

President's Medal of University of Texas–Houston Health Science Center (first recipient), 1987

City Builder Award, presented by the South Main Center Association, 1988

John P. McGovern Day, Resolution passed by County Commissioners Court, Harris County, Texas, September 13, 1988

John P. McGovern Day, proclamation signed by Kathryn J. Whitmire, Mayor of the City of Houston, October 17, 1988

Honorary Life Member, University of Texas Medical Branch at Galveston, declared by Alumni Association, 1988

Distinguished Service Award for "Outstanding Contributions to the Behavioral Sciences and the Prevention of Alcoholism and Drug Abuse," Alcohol and Drug Abuse Problems Association of North America, 1988

Caring for America Award ("for outstanding contributions to the American public"), National Federation of Republican Women, 1988
Special Award for Meritorious Service, Board of Trustees, American Medical Association, 1988
Surgeon General's Medallion, awarded by C. Everett Koop, MD, ScD., Surgeon General of the United States, 1989
Distinguished Service Award, International Council on Alcohol and Addictions, 1989
Outstanding Alumnus Award, Phi Beta Kappa Alumni of Greater Houston, 1991
First Cultural Heritage Award, University of Texas Institute of Texan Culture at San Antonio, 1991
Community Spirit Award, Volunteers of America, 1991
American Eagle Award, Cancer Fighters of Houston, 1991
Appreciation Award, Texas Neurofibromatosis Foundation, 1991
First Honorary Partner, Points of Light Campaign, Volunteer Center, 1991
Caring Spirit Award, Institute of Religion, Houston, Texas, 1992
Annual Synergy Award, The Park People, 1995
20th Anniversary Founders Award, South Main Center Association, Houston, 1996
Maurice Hirsh Award for Philanthropy, National Society of Fundraising Executives, Greater Houston Chapter, 1997
Rotary Club Fellow, 2000 (member from 1983)
Founders Award (one of three original founders), Houston Museum District, 2000
Lifetime of Service Award, Cancer League of Houston, 2000
Distinguished Citizen Award, Rotary Club of Houston, 2001
Laura Lee Blanton Community Spirit Award, Hospice at the Texas Medical Center, 2001
Mayor's Proud Partners 2001 Award for the John P. McGovern's Children's Zoo, Keep Houston Beautiful Campaign
The GHPA President's Award, 2001 Good Brick Awards, Greater Houston Preservation Alliance, 2002
Mary Jo Peckham Award, Assistance League of Houston, 2002
Honoree, *Gala de Paris,* Harris County Medical Society Alliance Philanthropic Fund, Houston, 2002
Lifetime of Achievement Award inaugural honoree, Aspiring Youth Organization, Houston, 2002

Sustaining Presence Award, Interfaith CarePartners, Houston, 2003
Honoree, Baylor Women's Faculty Club of Baylor College of Medicine, 2003
2003 President's Award, Texas Association of Museums, 2003
First Honoree, Inaugural Gala, John P. McGovern Museum of Health & Medical Science, 2003
Leadership Award, The Park People, Houston, 2003
Green Leaf Award, Houston Arboretum & Nature Center, 2003
Houston Hall of Fame, inducted 2003
Distinguished Service Award, Cosmos Club, Washington, DC, 2003
Ima Hogg Award, Mental Health Association of Harris County, Houston, 2004
John P. McGovern Lifetime Achievement Award, first recipient, American Lung Association of Texas–Houston & Southeast Region, 2004
Outstanding Individual Award, Houston Symphony League, 2006

FOREIGN AWARDS AND DECORATIONS

Honorary Member, Sociedad de Alergia y Ciencias Afines (Mexico), 1968
Honorary Member, La Sociedad Mexicana de Alergia e Immunología, A.C. (Mexico), 1968
Honorary Member, Canadian Allergy Society, 1968
Gold Medal Award "for meritorious and outstanding contributions in the field of pediatric allergy," twelfth International Congress of Pediatrics, Mexico City, 1968
Honorary Member, Asociatión Argentina de Alergia (Venezuela), 1972
Diploma de Honor al Mérito, República de Venezuela, "por su contribución as avance de las Ciencias Médicas y por su colaboración para con los venezolanos," 1973
Honorary Member, Groupement des allergologistes et immunologistes de langues latines, Paris, France, 1973–1984
Honorary Fellow, Royal College of Physicians (FRCP), London, 1984
Honorary Life President, Friends of 13 Norham Gardens, University of Oxford, Oxford, England, 1986
Statue of Responsibility Award, awarded by the Institute of Logotherapy at the sixth World Congress of Logotherapy, Buenos Aires, Argentina, 1987
Royal Medallion of the Polar Star, awarded by the King of Sweden, 1988

Auspiciador Award, Universidad del Pacífico, Lima, Perú, 1988
Heráldica de Cristóbal Colón, awarded by the President of the Dominican Republic, 1988
Miguel Alemán Award, Mexico, 1988
L'Ordre National du Mérite, awarded by President Mitterrand of France, 1988
Knighted in the Royal Order of San Miguel de Ala, Portugal, 1988
Decorated Comendador in La Orden Nacional José Matías Delgado, by Ing. José Napoleón Duarte, President of the Republic of El Salvador, 1988
Decorated Grado Comendador on Orden de Mayo al Mérito by Raúl Ricardo Alfonsín, President of the Republic of Argentina, 1988
Honorary Professor at the Universidad del Pacífico, invested by Rector Estuardo Loazya, Lima, Perú, 1988
Award of Distinction, awarded by the Mayor of Manila, 1989
The K. Attaturk Gold Medal Distinguished Service Award, the first awarded to an American citizen by the Government of Turkey, 1989
Distinguished Service Award, Pan American Medical Association, 1989

Appendix B

Editorial Appointments

Academic Achievement
Editorial Board, 1967–1975

ALERGIA, Iberoamerican Review of Allergy
Associate Editor, 1972–1982

Annals of Allergy: Official Journal of the American College of Allergy, Asthma & Immunology
Editorial Board, 1959–1965
Associate Editor, 1965–1980
Chairman, Editorial Board, 1980–1990

American Lecture Series in Allergy and Immunology
Editor, 1964–1980

Bulletin of the Medical Library Association
Consulting Editor, 1986–1989

Chronic Disease Management
Editorial Advisory Board, 1967–1974

Chronobiology International
Editorial Board, 1984–1990

The Classics of Medicine Library
Editorial Advisory Board, 1978

Clinical Proceedings of Children's Hospital of the District of Columbia, Washington, DC
Associate Editor, 1950–1954

Consultant
Editorial Advisory Board, 1970–1984

Emergency Medicine
Editorial Advisory Board, 1971–1986

Forum on Medicine (Official Journal of the American College of Physicians)
Editorial Advisory Board, 1978–1981

Geriatrics
Editorial Board, 1974–1978

Headache
Associate Editor, 1961–1976

Houston Medical Journal
Editorial Board, Senior Editorial Consultant, 1985–1994

The Journal of Asthma Research
Associate Editor, 1963–1980

The Journal of School Health (Official Journal of the American School Health Association)
Editorial Board, 1973–1976
Associate Editor, 1977–1980

The Letter of the International Correspondence Society of America
Editorial Board, 1961–1981

Medical Communications (Official Journal of the American Medical Writers Association)
Editorial Board, 1984–1987

Newsletter, Chapter-at-Large, Sigma Xi, Scientific Research Society
Editor, 1970–1972

Psychosomatics
Advisory Editor (Allergy), 1962–1972

Review of Allergy
Contributing Editor, 1959–1965

Texas Medicine
Editorial Consultant, 1965–1979

Appendix C

Professorships, Facilities, and Endowed Programs Named for McGovern

John P. McGovern, MD, Scholarship, Alpha Epsilon Delta (National Premedical Honor Society), University of Houston, 1976

John P. McGovern Award (highest award given annually), Texas School Health Association, 1977

John P. McGovern, MD, Scholarship Award, Eta Sigma Gamma (National Professional Health Science Honorary), 1979

John P. McGovern Phi Beta Kappa Alumni of Greater Houston Scholarship, 1980

John P. McGovern Visiting Professor, University of Texas-Houston Health Science Center, 1981–1996

John P. McGovern Award Lectureship in Allied Health Sciences, University of Texas–Houston Health Science Center, 1982

John P. McGovern History of Medicine Collection (John P. McGovern Historical Collections and Research Center), Houston Academy of Medicine–Texas Medical Center Library, 1982

John P. McGovern, MD, Award for Excellence in Psychiatry (undergraduate medical curriculum), Baylor College of Medicine, 1983

John P. McGovern Award Lectureship on the Medical Humanities, University of Texas Medical Branch at Galveston, 1982

John P. McGovern Award Lectureship in Medical Communication, Medical Library Association, 1983

John P. McGovern Award Lectureship in Allergy and Immunology, American College of Allergy, Asthma & Immunology, 1983

John P. McGovern Award Lectureship in Information and Communication, American Medical Writers Association, Southwest Chapter, 1983

John P. McGovern Award Lectureship in Continuing Education, Baylor College of Medicine, 1983–1997

John P. McGovern Award Lectureship in Health Science, Ball State University, 1983

John P. McGovern Award Lectureship on Science and Society, Sigma Xi, Research Society, 1983

John P. McGovern Award Lectureship in Communication, University of Texas at Austin, 1983–1999

John P. McGovern Award Lecture, American Osler Society, 1983

John P. McGovern Award Medal of the American Medical Writers Association, 1984

John P. McGovern Regents Professorship in Medical Journalism, University of Texas at Austin, 1984–1998

John P. McGovern Award Lectureship in School Health, American School Health Association, 1984

John P. McGovern Centennial Award Lectureship in Communication, University of Texas at Austin, 1984–1998

John P. McGovern, MD Scholarship, Galveston College, 1984

John P. McGovern Outstanding Teacher Award, University of Texas–Houston Medical School, 1984

John P. McGovern Outstanding Teacher Award, University of Texas–Houston Graduate School of Biomedical Sciences, 1984

John P. McGovern Outstanding Teacher Award, University of Texas–Houston School of Nursing, 1984

John P. McGovern Outstanding Teacher Award, University of Texas–Houston School of Allied Health Sciences, 1984

John P. McGovern Outstanding Teacher Award, University of Texas–Houston Dental Branch, 1984

John P. McGovern Outstanding Teacher Award, University of Texas–Houston School of Public Health, 1984

John P. McGovern Scholarship, Pi Kappa Alpha, 1984

John P. McGovern Allergy Society, founded by McGovern's colleagues and former fellows at the 42nd Annual Congress of the American College of Allergy, Asthma & Immunology, 1986

John P. McGovern Clinical Scholars Program, School of Nursing, University of Texas–Houston Health Science Center, 1986

John P. McGovern Award Lectureship in the Arts and Humanities, Cosmos Club, Washington, DC, 1986

John P. McGovern Award Lectureship in Science, Cosmos Club, Washington, DC, 1986

John P. McGovern Award Lectureship in Literature, Cosmos Club, Washington, DC, 1986

John P. McGovern Hall of Medical History, Ashbel Smith Building, University of Texas Medical Branch at Galveston, 1986

John P. McGovern Award for Distinguished Service in the Health Sciences, Association of Academic Health Centers, Washington, DC, 1988

McGovern Mammal Marina dedicated in honor of Dr. and Mrs. John P. McGovern, Houston Zoological Gardens, 1988

Dr. and Mrs. John P. McGovern Hall of Minerals, Houston Museum of Natural Science, 1988–1996

John P. McGovern Outstanding Premedical Student Award, Rice University, 1988

John P. McGovern Award in the Behavioral Sciences, the American Association for the Advancement of Science, 1988

John P. McGovern Award in Behavioral Science, the Smithsonian Institution, 1988

John P. McGovern Centennial Distinguished Professorship in Family Medicine (certified in addiction medicine), University of Texas Medical Branch at Galveston, 1990

McGovern Drug and Alcohol Three-Quarter Way House, Volunteers of American-Houston, Inc., 1990

John P. McGovern Award Lectureship, Association for Medical Education and Research in Substance Abuse, 1991

John P. McGovern Annual Award, American Association of Colleges of Nursing, 1991

John P. McGovern Annual Seminar in Health, Education and Research, Women's Fund for HER, 1991

John P. McGovern Award Lectureship in the Art and Science of Medicine, Texas A&M University College of Medicine, 1993

John P. McGovern Annual Award Lectureship in the Medical Humanities, the C. Everett Koop Institute at Dartmouth, 1993

John P. McGovern Compleat Physician Award, Houston Academy of Medicine, 1993

John P. McGovern Annual Award Lectureship—Humanities in Medicine, Yale University School of Medicine, 1993

John P. McGovern Award Lectureship in the Art and Science of Medicine, Duke University, 1995

John P. McGovern Award Lectureship in Health Promotion, Center for Health Promotion and Prevention Research, School of Public Health, University of Texas–Houston Health Science Center, 1995

John P. McGovern Professorship in Nursing, School of Nursing, University of Texas–Houston Health Science Center, 1996–1998

John P. McGovern Professorship in Health Promotion, School of Public Health, University of Texas–Houston Health Science Center, 1996

John P. McGovern Building–Museum of Health & Medical Science, Houston, 1996

McGovern Theater, Museum of Health & Medical Science, Houston, 1996

John P. McGovern Outstanding Pre-Medical Student Award, Rice University, Houston, 1996

Dr. and Mrs. John P. McGovern Pigmy Hippo Habitat Exhibit, Houston Zoological Gardens, 1996

Dr. and Mrs. John P. McGovern Gallery, Hall of Minerals, Houston Museum of Natural Science, 1996

John P. McGovern Historical Collections and Research Center, Houston Academy of Medicine–Texas Medical Center Library, 1996

Dr. and Mrs. John P. McGovern Amazon Rainforest Wing, Kipp Aquarium, Houston Zoological Gardens, 1996

John P. McGovern Award Lectureship in the History of Medicine, Harvard University Medical School, 1996

John P. McGovern, MD Distinguished Professorship in Ophthalmology, School of Medicine, University of Texas–Houston Health Science Center, 1997

John P. McGovern Student Awards, Graduate School of Biomedical Sciences, University of Texas–Houston Health Science Center, 1997

John P. McGovern Annual Award on Addiction and Society, American Society of Addiction Medicine, 1997

John P. McGovern Distinguished Professorship in Nursing, School of Nursing, University of Texas–Houston Health Science Center, 1998

John P. McGovern Hall of the Americas, Houston Museum of Natural Science, 1998

John P. McGovern Award Lectureship in the Art and Science of Medicine, Baylor College of Medicine, 1998

John P. McGovern Professorship in Health and Medical Science Communication, College of Communication, University of Texas at Austin, 1998 (formerly John P. McGovern Regents Professorship in Health Communication)

John P. McGovern Professorship in Addiction Nursing, School of Nursing, University of Texas–Houston Health Science Center, 1998

McGovern Lake, Hermann Park, Houston, 1998

John P. McGovern Children's Zoo, Houston Zoological Gardens, 1998

John P. McGovern Award Lectureship in Family, Health, and Family Values, College of Liberal Arts and Social Sciences, University of Houston, 1999 (formerly College of Humanities, Fine Arts and Communication)

McGovern Lecture on Medical Chronobiology and Chronotherapeutics, American Association for Medical Chronobiology and Chronotherapeutics, 1999

John P. McGovern, MD Visitors Gallery, University of Texas–M. D. Anderson Cancer Center, 1999

John P. McGovern Award Lectureship in Health Communication, University of Texas at Austin, 1999

John P. McGovern Veterans Health Care and Service Center, DeGeorge at Union Station, Houston, 1999

McGovern-Davison Children's Health Center, Duke University Medical Center, 2000

John P. McGovern Award, Alcohol and Drug Abuse Women's Center, Galveston, 2000

John P. McGovern Award Lectureship in Oslerian Medicine, Johns Hopkins University, 2000

Osler-McGovern Centre, 13 Norham Gardens, Green College, Oxford University, 2000

John P. McGovern Award in the History and Philosophy of Medicine, Graduate School of Biomedical Sciences, University of Texas–Houston Health Science Center, 2001

John P. McGovern Award Lectureship in the History and Philosophy of

Medicine, History of Medicine Society, Baylor College of Medicine, 2000

John P. McGovern Annual Award Lectureship in Oslerian Medicine, Green College, Oxford University, 2000 (now Green Templeton College)

John P. McGovern Professorship in the Healing Practices of Nursing, University of Texas Medical Branch at Galveston, 2000

John P. McGovern, MD Presidential Portrait Gallery and Charters of Freedom Hall, Ronald Reagan Library, Simi Valley, California, 2001

John P. McGovern Graduate School of Biomedical Sciences Endowed Professorship, Graduate School of Biomedical Sciences, University of Texas Health Science Center at Houston, 2001

John P. McGovern, MD Center for Environmental and Regulatory Affairs, National Center for Public Policy Research, Washington, DC, 2001

John P. McGovern Kids Hall, Children's Museum of Houston, 2001

The Bryant Boutwell, DrPH and John P. McGovern, MD Scholarship for Medical Students from Disadvantaged Backgrounds at the University of Texas Medical School at Houston, 2001

John P. McGovern Library, Cosmos Club, Washington, DC, 2002

John P. McGovern Museum of Health and Science, Houston, 2002

John P. McGovern/Texas Medical Center Commons, Texas Medical Center, Houston, 2002

John P. McGovern Campus Park, Houston, 2002

John P. McGovern/Stella Link Library, Houston, 2002

John P. McGovern Professorship in Oslerian Medicine, the Medical School, University of Texas Health Science Center at Houston, 2003

John P. and Kathrine G. McGovern Gardens, John P. McGovern/Texas Medical Center Commons, Texas Medical Center, Houston 2003

John P. McGovern Champion of Health Award, Texas Medical Association Foundation, Austin, 2004

John P. McGovern Asthma Education Program, American Lung Association of Texas, Houston & Southeast Region Asthma School Program, 2004

John P. McGovern Lifetime Achievement Award, American Lung Association of Texas, Houston & Southeast Region, 2004.

John P. McGovern, MD Community Sports and Recreation Building, Community Family Centers, Houston, 2004

John P. McGovern Campus, Texas Medical Center (Holcombe site), Houston, 2004

John P. McGovern Lifetime Service Award, the Cancer League, Houston, 2004

John P. McGovern, MD Center for Health, Humanities, and the Human Spirit, at the Medical School, University of Texas Health Science Center at Houston, 2005 (in 2010 renamed McGovern Center for Humanities and Ethics)

John P. McGovern Children's Discovery Area, Armand Bayou Nature Center, Houston, 2005

John P. McGovern Distinguished Professorship in Oslerian Medicine, University of Texas Medical Branch at Galveston, 2007

Notes

Abbreviations

HAM-TMC—Houston Academy of Medicine–Texas Medical Center
JPM—John P. McGovern
JPM-HC—John P. McGovern Historical Collections and Research Center, Texas Medical Center Library, Houston
Papers—John P. McGovern Papers at John P. McGovern Historical Collections and Research Center, Texas Medical Center Library, Houston

Introduction

1. *Appreciations, Reminiscences and Tributes Honoring John P. McGovern,* ed. Gilbert D. Barkin et al. (Houston: Health Sciences Institute, 1980).

2. JPM to Bryant Boutwell, November 29, 1994, Papers, MS 115, Box 6: Office Files, Books and Publications, Folder 6: B. Boutwell; Boylan, Michael.

3. Dale Lezon and Todd Ackerman, "Doctor Became Known for Giving," *Houston Chronicle,* June 1, 2007.

4. Finding Aid for the John P. McGovern Papers, Papers, MS 115.

5. Grant Taylor, introduction to *Appreciations,* 5.

Chapter One

1. Michael Bliss, *The Discovery of Insulin* (Chicago: University of Chicago Press, 2007).

2. Francis McGovern to JPM, June 29, 1921, Papers, MS 115, Box: Personal Correspondence 4, Folder 3: Special letter on Jack's birth.

3. Ann Gallagher to JPM, no date, Papers, MS 115, Box: Personal Correspondence 4, Folder 8: JPM Correspondence.

4. Wedding Announcement of Lottie Brown and Dr. Francis McGovern, October 13, 1918, Papers, MS 115, Box: McGovern Personal 5, Folder 6: Lottie Brown McGovern Photographs.

5. Thomas E. Mahoney, contribution to *Appreciations,* 114 (see intro., n. 1).

6. Constance McLaughlin Green, *Washington: A History of the Capital, 1800–1950* (Princeton: Princeton University Press, 1962), 380.

7. Ibid., 377.

8. Robert S. McElvaine, *The Great Depression: America 1929–1941* (New York: Random House, 1993), Kindle edition.

9. Paul Dickson and Thomas B. Allen, *The Bonus Army: An American Epic* (New York: Walker, 2004).

10. Green, *Washington: A History,* 373.

11. Shelby Hodge, "A Gift for Giving: Heritage of Generosity Sets Houston Doctor on Lifelong Philanthropic Path," *Houston Chronicle,* August 25, 1996.

12. Theodore Wiprud, "Francis Xavier McGovern, M.D., F.A.C.S. (1893–1951)," *Medical Annals of the District of Columbia* 20, no. 10 (1951): 577–78.

13. "Hospital Center History," MedStar Washington Hospital Center, last modified January 25, 2012, http://www.whcenter.org/body.cfm?id=555916.

14. Washington Hospital Center Act, Public Law 648, 79th Congress, Chapter 803, 2nd Session, S. 223 (August 7, 1946).

15. Erik Larson, *In the Garden of Beasts: Love, Terror, and an American Family in Hitler's Berlin* (New York: Crown, 2011), Kindle edition.

16. Philippine Independence Act, Public Law 73–127, 48 Stat. 456 (March 24, 1934).

17. Eleanor D. Tydings to Francis McGovern, July 31, 1946, Papers, MS 115, Box: Personal Correspondence 4, Folder 17: F. X. McGovern Various Documents.

18. "Mac McGovern, Washingtonian of the Week," *Washington Post,* January 3, 1941.

19. Wiprud, "Francis Xavier McGovern," 577–78.

20. Ibid.

21. A. Ziegler McPherson, contribution to *Appreciations,* 30.

22. JPM to Lottie Brown, October 5, 1964, Papers, MS 115, Box: Personal Correspondence 4, Folder 7: Jack's Letters to Mother 1960–1978.

23. Andrea Barrett, *Ship Fever* (New York: Norton, 1996), 159–60.

24. Susan Campbell Bartoletti, *Black Potatoes: The Story of the Great Irish Famine, 1845–1850* (Boston: Houghton Mifflin, 2001), 1.

25. Ibid., 15.

26. Kerby Miller, *Emigrants and Exiles: Ireland and the Irish Exodus to North America* (New York: Oxford University Press, 1985), 569.

27. Bartoletti, *Black Potatoes,* 7.

28. Ann Gallagher to JPM, no date, Papers, MS 115, Box: Personal Correspondence 4, Folder 8: JPM Correspondence.

29. John Fahrnkoff, District of Columbia naturalization papers certifying U.S. citizenship, May 27, 1862, Papers, MS 115, Box 6, Folder: Personal.

30. Hodge, "A Gift for Giving."

31. JPM, personal conversation with the author, April 2000.

32. Bank book belonging to JPM, May 27, 1929, Papers, MS 115, Box: Personal Correspondence 4, Folder: Personal Correspondence.

33. JPM to Mary Brown, July 12, 1929, Papers, MS 115, Box: Personal Correspondence 4, Folder 13: Jack to Grandmother Brown.

34. JPM dictation to Julia Mitchell, 1993, 3, Papers, MS 115, Box: Personal 1, Folder: Helen Hayes.

35. Helen Hayes, *On Reflection: An Autobiography* (New York: M. Evans, 1968), 20.

36. Ibid., 19.

37. Ibid., 32.

38. Ibid., 28–30.

39. Ibid., 33.

40. Ibid.

41. Brad Snyder, *Beyond the Shadow of the Senators* (New York: McGraw-Hill, 2004), 4.

42. JPM dictation to Julia Mitchell, 1993, 3.

43. Helen Hayes, contribution to *Appreciations*, 262.

44. Robert S. McElvaine, *The Great Depression.*

45. Green, *Washington: A History*, 338–39.

46. Ibid., 341.

47. Ibid., 342.

48. Ibid., 346.

49. "Origins," a history of Washington schools written by high school students, 29, Papers, MS 115, Series: McGovern Personal, Box 6.

50. Ibid., 29–30.

51. Ibid., 30.

52. Ibid., 30–31.

53. Woodrow Wilson High School Yearbook, 6.

54. "Humanism in Medicine and in Life: A Profile of John P. McGovern, MD," *Houston Review of History and Culture* 2, no. 1 (Fall 2004): 34. Information for this profile article came from a series of interviews with Dr. McGovern by William H. Kellar during the spring of 2000.

55. Woodrow Wilson High School Yearbook, 6.

56. Jon Meacham, "The American Dream Has Seen Better Days—Much Better," *Time*, July 2, 2012.

57. JPM, personal conversation with the author, February 1998.

58. Alice Schroeder, *The Snowball: Warren Buffett and the Business of Life* (New York: Bantam, 2009), Kindle edition.

59. Woodrow Wilson High School Yearbook, 6.

60. Schroeder, *The Snowball*, Kindle edition.

61. JPM, "Medicine as a Vocation," junior high school paper, 6, undated, Papers, MS 115, Box: Personal 6, Folder: Misc.

Chapter Two

1. Wilburt C. Davison, “Memories of Sir William Osler,” in *William Osler Commemorative Issue,* special issue, *Journal of the American Medical Association* 210, no. 12 (December 22, 1969): 2219–22.

2. Jay M. Arena, MD, “The Wrecker Was a Builder,” in *The Davison Issue,* special issue, *Davison Alumni Publications* 8, no. 5B (July 1968): 6–10.

3. JPM to Wilburt Davison, November 11, 1966, Papers, MS 115, Box: Davison 1, Folder: Davison Correspondence with McGovern 1960–1972.

4. JPM tribute to Dean Davison, Papers, MS 115, Box: Davison 4, Folder 7: Davison Memorial. This address was delivered during Wilburt Davison's memorial service held at the Duke Chapel on November 17, 1972.

5. Harvey Cushing, *The Life of Sir William Osler* (London: Oxford University Press, 1940), 30–31.

6. Ibid., 222.

7. “What's With That Pesky ‘S’?” Johns Hopkins Medicine, accessed February 18, 2013, http://www.hopkinsmedicine.org/about/history/history1.html.

8. Michael Bliss, *William Osler: A Life in Medicine* (New York: Oxford University Press, 1999), 200.

9. Ibid., 205.

10. William Osler, *Aequanimitas, with Other Addresses to Medical Students, Nurses, and Practitioners of Medicine,* 3rd ed. (Philadelphia: Blakiston, 1932), 390.

11. William Osler, “Address to the Students of the Albany Medical College,” *Albany Medical Annual* 20 (1899): 307–9.

12. William Osler, “The Reserves of Life,” *St. Mary's Hospital Gazette* 13 (1907): 95–98.

13. William Feindel, Elizabeth Maloney, and Pamela Miller, eds., *Sir William Osler: The Man and His Books* (Montreal: Osler Library of the History of Medicine, McGill University, 2011): 16.

14. Ibid., vii.

15. Cushing, *The Life of Sir William Osler,* 357–58.

16. Anne Bennett Swingle, “The Rockefeller Chronicle,” *Hopkins Medical News* (Fall 2002), accessed January 6, 2013, http://www.hopkinsmedicine.org/hmn/F02/annals.html.

17. Bliss, *William Osler: A Life in Medicine,* 506.

18. E. H. Bensley and D. G. Bates, “Sir William Osler's Autobiographical Notes,” *Bulletin of the History of Medicine* 50 (1976): 596–618.

19. Richard L. Golden, “William Osler at 150: An Overview of a Life,” *Journal of the American Medical Association* 282, no. 23 (December 15, 1999): 2253.

20. P. H. Starling, “The Case of Edward Revere Osler,” *Journal of the Royal Army Medical Corps* 149 (2003): 27–29.

21. Ibid.

22. Ibid.

23. Grace Osler to Wilburt Davison, May 7, 1918, Papers, MS 115, Box: Davison 4, Folder: Wilburt C. Davison Various.

24. Cushing, *The Life of Sir William Osler,* 1366.

25. Davison, "Memories of Sir William Osler," 2219.

26. Jay M. Arena and JPM, eds., *Davison of Duke: His Reminiscences* (Durham: Duke University Press, 1980), 33.

27. Davison, "Memories of Sir William Osler," 2219.

28. Ibid., 2219–20.

29. William Osler, *Aequanimitas,* 104.

30. Davison, "Memories of Sir William Osler," 2220.

31. Arena, *Davison of Duke,* 58.

32. Jay M. Arena, "Duke's Mixture: Davison's Saga," *Clinical Pediatrician* 7, no. 4 (April 1968): 232–37.

33. Jay M. Arena, "Wilburt Cornell Davison: He Built a Medical School of Stone—and Left It Marble," *American Journal of Diseases of Children* 124 (September 1972): 338.

34. Herbert Swick, e-mail message to the author, May 17, 2012.

35. Wilburt C. Davison to JPM, May 28, 1961, Papers, MS 115, Series 7, Box 1, Folder 1.1: Correspondence with Davison 1945–1962.

36. Wilburt C. Davison, "History of Duke University Medical Center (1892–1960)," unpublished 3rd draft (December 31, 1965), 4a, n2, Papers, MS 115, Box: Davison 3, Folder 1: Davison—Origins of the Duke Medical Library 1962; History of Duke University Medical Center 1966.

37. Thomas Neville Bonner, *Iconoclast: Abraham Flexner and a Life in Learning* (Baltimore: Johns Hopkins University Press, 2002), 21.

38. Davison, "History of Duke University Medical Center (1892–1960)," 3, Papers, MS 115, Box: Davison 3, Folder 1: Davison—Origins of the Duke Medical Library 1962; History of Duke University Medical Center 1966.

39. Arena, *Davison of Duke,* 107.

40. Ibid.

41. Davison, "History of Duke University Medical Center (1892–1960)," 11a.

42. Arena, *Davison of Duke,* 100–101.

43. Davison, "Memories of Sir William Osler," 2220.

44. William Osler, "The Functions of a State Faculty," *Maryland Medical Journal* 37 (May 15, 1897): 73–77.

45. Arena, *Davison of Duke,* 126.

46. Wilburt C. Davison, interview by J. E. Markee, transcript of a video titled *Origins of the Duke Hospital Medical Library* (November 26, 1962), 2, in Papers, MS 115, Box: Davison 3, Folder 1: Davison—Origins of the Duke Medical Library 1962; History of Duke University Medical Center 1966.

47. Davison, "History of Duke University Medical Center," 6.

48. Ibid.

49. Arena, *Davison of Duke,* 111.

50. Davison, "History of Duke University Medical Center," 11.

51. Ibid., 9.

52. William H. Welch, "Changing Viewpoints in Medical Education," *Southern Medical Journal* 24 (1931): 1121–24.

53. H. J. Herring to JPM, June 27, 1939, Papers, MS 115, Box: Scrapbook 1, 1939–1962, Folder 1: 1939.

54. Jay Maxwell, contribution to *Appreciations,* 28 (see intro., n. 1).

55. JPM to Francis McGovern, September 18, 1939, Papers, MS 115, Box: Personal Correspondence 5, Folder 5: Jack's Letters to Mother and Dad 1939–1950.

56. Woodrow Wilson High School Yearbook 6 (see chap. 1, n. 53).

57. JPM to Francis McGovern, September 18, 1939, Papers, MS 115, Box: Personal Correspondence 5, Folder 5: Jack's Letters to Mother and Dad 1939–1950.

58. Ibid., October 21, 1939.

59. Ibid.

60. JPM to Lottie McGovern, March 22, 1940, Papers, MS 115, Box: Personal Correspondence 5, Folder 5: Jack's Letters to Mother and Dad 1939–1950.

61. JPM, telephone conversation with Bryant Boutwell, November 1997.

62. *The Duke Aesculapian 1966* (Durham: Duke University Medical Center), 116, Papers, MS 115, Box: McGovern Personal 6.

63. Richard M. Paddison, contribution to *Appreciations,* 32.

64. JPM to Francis McGovern, Sunday morning 1944 (undated), Papers, MS 115, Box: Personal Correspondence 4, Folder 5: Letters to Mother and Dad, 1939–1950.

65. A. Ziegler McPherson, contribution to *Appreciations,* 30–31.

66. JPM to Francis McGovern and Lottie Brown, April 10, 1943, Papers, MS 115, Box: Personal Correspondence 4, Folder 5: Letters to Mother and Dad, 1939–1950.

67. Arena, *Davison of Duke,* 108.

68. JPM to Francis McGovern and Lottie Brown, April 13, 1944, Papers, MS 115, Box: Personal Correspondence 4, Folder 5: Letters to Mother and Dad, 1939–1950.

69. Ibid.

70. Francis McGovern to JPM, April 25, 1943, Papers, MS 115, Box: Personal Correspondence 4, Folder 2: Father's letters to Jack 1943, 1944.

71. Sue Ann Gardner, "Gail Borden," *Faculty Publications, UNL Libraries* (1999), http://digitalcommons.unl.edu/libraryscience/110.

72. Ibid.

73. Joe B. Frantz, *Gail Borden: Dairyman to a Nation* (Norman: University of Oklahoma Press, 1951).

74. "New Article of Food—Meat Biscuit," *Scientific American* 5, no. 27 (March 23, 1850): 213.

75. "Pertussis (Whooping Cough)—What you need to know," Centers for Disease Control and Prevention, last modified January 9, 2013, http://www.cdc.gov/Features/Pertussis/.

76. Jules Bordet and Octave Gengou, "Le Microbe de las Coqueluche," *Annales de l'Institut Pasteur* 20 (1906): 731–41.

77. "Pertussis (Whooping Cough)."

78. Grant Taylor, introduction to *Appreciations,* 6.

79. Hilda Pope Willett, contribution to *Appreciations,* 52–54.

80. Francis McGovern to JPM, August 19, 1944, Papers, MS 115, Box: Personal Correspondence 4, Folder 2: Father's letters to Jack 1943, 1944.

81. Donna Gordon Blankinship, "Whooping Cough Epidemic Declared in Washington State," *Houston Chronicle,* May 10, 2012.

82. Francis McGovern to JPM, December 8, 1944, Papers, MS 115, Box: Personal Correspondence 4, Folder 2: Father's letters to Jack 1943, 1944.

83 Kathrine G. McGovern, interview by the author, August 18, 2010.

84. JPM to Francis McGovern and Lottie Brown, October 30, 1943, John P. McGovern papers, MS 115, Box: Personal Correspondence 4, Folder 5: Jack's Letters to Mother and Dad 1939–1950.

85. Francis McGovern to JPM, April 22, 1945, Papers, MS 115, Box: Personal Correspondence 4, Folder 1: Father's Letters to Jack 1943–1944.

86. Ibid., May 20, 1945, Papers, MS 115, Box: Personal Correspondence 4, Folder 1: Father's letters to Jack 1945–1948.

87. JPM to Francis McGovern, May 25, 1944, Papers, MS 115, Box: Personal Correspondence 4, Folder 5: Letters to Mother and Dad, 1939–1950.

88. Francis McGovern to JPM, January 9, 1944, Papers, MS 115, Box: Personal Correspondence 4, Folder 1: Father's Letters to Jack 1943–1944.

89. A. C. Gray to Francis McGovern, October 2, 1945, Papers, MS 115, Box: Personal Correspondence 4, Folder 17: Letters re: resignation of F. X. McGovern; other correspondence of F. X.

90. JPM to Francis McGovern and Lottie Brown, April 10, 1943, Papers, MS 115, Box: Personal Correspondence 4, Folder 5: Letters to Mother and Dad, 1939–1950.

91. JPM, Oral History interview by Charles T. Morrissey, June 25, 1997, Baylor College of Medicine, Houston, Texas, Papers, MS 115, Series 7, Box: 16, Folder: 17 Oral History Transcript—1998.

92. Francis McGovern to JPM, May 30, 1946, Papers, MS 115, Box: Personal Correspondence 4, Folder 1: Father's letters to Jack 1945–1948.

93. Ibid., May 20, 1945, Papers, MS 115, Box: Personal Correspondence 4, Folder 1: Father's letters to Jack 1945–1948.

94. Francis McGovern to JPM, August 19, 1946, Papers, MS 115, Box: Personal Correspondence 4, Folder 1: Father's letters to Jack 1945–1948.

95. Wiprud, "Francis Xavier McGovern," 577–78.

96. Wilburt C. Davison to Lottie Brown, August 7, 1951, Papers, MS 115, Series 7, Box 1, Folder 1.1: Correspondence with Davison 1945–1962.

97. JPM to Lottie Brown, October 30, 1968, Papers, MS 115, Box: Personal Correspondence 4, Folder 6: Jack's letters to Mother 1960–1978.

98. Jeremiah A. Barondess, "A Brief History of Mentoring," *Transactions of the American Clinical Climatological Association* 106 (1995): 1–24.

99. Wilburt C. Davison, "The Basis of Sir William Osler's Influence on Medicine," *Annals of Allergy* 27 (August 1969): 366–72.

Chapter Three

1. William S. Thayer, "The Chief: Remarks to the First Graduating Class of the Medical Department of Duke University on the Occasion of the Planting of a Sprig of Ivy from 13, Norham Gardens," *New England Journal of Medicine* 207, no. 13 (September 29, 1932): 563–70.

2. Denis M. O'Day and Mary R. Ladden, "The Influence of Derrick T. Vail, Sr., MD, and Edward M. Jackson, MD, on the Creation of the American Board of Ophthalmology and the Specialist Board System in the United States," *Archives of Ophthalmology* 130, no. 2 (2012): 224–32.

3. Rosemary Stevens, *American Medicine and the Public Interest: A History of Specialization* (Berkeley: University of California Press, 1998).

4. "Higher Standards Are the Foundation for Better Care," American Board of Medical Specialties, accessed February 9, 2013, http://www.abms.org/About_ABMS/who_we_are.aspx.

5. JPM to Francis McGovern and Lottie Brown, April 13, 1944, Papers, MS 115, Box: Personal Correspondence 4, Folder 5: Letters to Mother and Dad, 1939–1950.

6. JPM to Francis McGovern, May 3, 1944, Papers, MS 115, Box: Personal Correspondence 4, Folder 5: Letters to Mother and Dad, 1939–1950.

7. JPM to Lottie Brown, March 7, 1970, Papers, MS 115, Box: Personal Correspondence 4, Folder 6: Jack's letters to Mother 1960–1978.

8. JPM, "Medicine as a Vocation" (see chap. 1, n. 61).

9. Ibid., 5.

10. JPM to parents, December 2, 1943, Papers, MS 115, Box: Personal Correspondence 4, Folder 5: Letters to Mother and Dad, 1939–1950.

11. Julia Q. Mitchell, interview by the author, August 25, 2010.

12. Grant Taylor, introduction to *Appreciations,* 7 (see intro., n. 1).

13. Ibid.

14. C. Becket Mahnke, "The Growth and Development of a Specialty: The History of Pediatrics," *Clinical Pediatrics* 39, no. 12 (Dec. 2000): 710.

15. B. Lee Ligon-Borden, "Abraham Jacobi, MD: Father of American Pediatrics and Advocate for Children's Health," *Seminars in Pediatric Infectious Diseases* 20, no. 3 (July 2003): 245.

16. Ibid., 247.

17. Lawrence M. Gartner, "Tribute to Abraham Jacobi: World Leader in Medicine and Medical Historian," *Breastfeeding Medicine* 1, no. 2 (July 10, 2006): 112–14.

18. Wilburt C. Davison, "Pediatric Profiles: John Howland (1873–1926)," *Journal of Pediatrics* 46 (April 1955): 473–86.

19. "Declines Harvard Offer: Dr. John Howland to Remain at Johns Hopkins," *New York Times*, May 29, 1921.

20. Daniel C. Darrow, "Grover Francis Powers and Pediatrics at Yale," *Yale Journal of Biology and Medicine* 24, no. 4 (February 1952): 243–51.

21. Grover F. Powers, "Dr. Winternitz and Pediatrics at Yale," *Yale Journal of Biology and Medicine* 22, no. 6 (July 1950): 715–18.

22. Howard A. Pearson, "History of the Department of Pediatrics Yale University School of Medicine," *Yale Journal of Biology and Medicine* 70, no. 3 (1997): 202.

23. Ibid., 203.

24. Ibid., 204.

25. Taylor, introduction to *Appreciations*, 7.

26. Pearson, "History of the Department of Pediatrics," 204.

27. Darrow, "Grover Francis Powers and Pediatrics at Yale," 243.

28. Grover F. Powers, "First Things First in Medicine," *Yale Journal of Biology and Medicine* 29, no. 1 (September 1956): 7–8.

29. Herman Yannet, "Education: A Pediatric Interne and Resident Training Program Integrated with a Training School for the Mentally Retarded," *Pediatrics* 20, no. 1 (1957): 139–42.

30. Francis McGovern to JPM, July 19, 1945, Papers, MS 115, Box: Personal 4, Folder 2: Father's Letters to Jack 1945–1948.

31. Ibid., December 8, 1944, Papers, MS 115, Box: Personal Correspondence 4, Folder 2: Father's letters to Jack 1943, 1944.

32. Ibid., August 15, 1945, Papers, MS 115, Box: Personal 4, Folder 2: Father's Letters to Jack 1945–1948.

33. JPM, personal conversation with the author, April 2000.

34. Taylor, introduction to *Appreciations*, 8.

35. Herman Yannet, contribution to *Appreciations*, 58. Readers may be interested in the 1947 publication Yannet refers to, which was titled "Asymmetric Spastic Infantile Cerebral Palsy" and was published by the *American Journal of Disabled Children* 74, no. 2 (1947): 121–29.

36. Wilburt C. Davison to JPM, November 16, 1945, Papers, MS 115, Series 7, Box 1, Folder 1: Correspondence with Davison 1945–1962.

37. JPM to Wilburt C. Davison, July 17, 1951, Papers, MS 115, Series 7, Box 1, Folder 1: Correspondence with Davison 1945–1962.

38. Mault M. Pomerantz, "History of Resectional Surgery for Tuberculosis and Other Mycobacterial Infections," *Chest Surgery Clinics of North America* 10, no. 1 (February 2000): 131–33.

39. That equilibrium has been defined in the Preamble to the Constitution of the World Health Organization as adopted by the International Health Conference, New York, June 19–22, 1946, signed on July 22, 1946 by the representatives of sixty-one states (*Official Records of the World Health Organization*, no. 2: 100) and entered into force on April 7, 1948.

40. Taylor, introduction to *Appreciations,* 9.

41. Edwin L. Kendig Jr., contribution to *Appreciations,* 67.

42. Taylor, introduction to *Appreciations,* 9.

43. JPM, "An Unusual Case of Hypersensitivity to Cold Complicated by Paroxysmal Diarrhea," *Journal of Allergy* 19, no. 6 (1948): 408–10.

44. JPM, Theodore J. Haywood, Orville C. Thomas, et al., *Handbook for the Allergic Patient,* McGovern Allergy Clinic, 1976.

45. Joseph L. Kochka to Francis McGovern, March 31, 1947, Papers, MS 115, Box: Personal Correspondence 4, Folder 17: Letters re: resignation of F. X. McGovern; other correspondence of F. X.

46. "National Veterans Wheelchair Games: History of the Games," United States Department of Veterans Affairs, accessed February 9, 2013, http://www.va.gov/opa/speceven/wcg/docs/history.asp.

47. Harry A Schweikert, "History of Wheelchair Basketball," *Paraplegia News* 8, no. 18 (May 1954): 8–10.

48. James A. Caddy, contribution to *Appreciations,* 72.

49. Helen Hayes to JPM, November 27, 1948, Papers, MS 115, Box: Personal Correspondence 1, Folder 17: Helen Hayes.

50. Bill Lee, "Queen of the American Merchant Marine," USS Westpoint Reunion Association, accessed February 9, 2013, http://www.usswestpoint.com./index.cfm?fuseaction=seastory&story=SSAmericaanabbreviatedhistory.htm.

51. Bill Lee, "America's Spies: Potential Impact on America—and the SS America," USS Westpoint Reunion Association, accessed February 9, 2013, http://www.usswestpoint.com/index.cfm?fuseaction=seastory&story=AMERICAsSpies.htm#LinkTarget_971.

52. Bill Lee, "Queen of the American Merchant Marine," USS Westpoint Reunion Association, accessed February 9, 2013, http://www.usswestpoint.com/index.cfm?fuseaction=seastory&story=SSAmericaanabbreviatedhistory.htm.

53. Michael Bliss, *William Osler: A Life in Medicine,* 506 (see chap. 2, n. 8).

54. *A Copy of the Last Will and Testament of Thomas Guy, Esq. with an Act for Incorporating the Executors of the Said Will* (London: Guy's Hospital, 1815).

55. Bliss, *William Osler: A Life in Medicine,* 68.

56. Arena, *Davison of Duke,* 63–64 (see chap. 2, n. 26).

57. JPM to Francis McGovern and Lottie Brown, March 21, 1949, Papers, MS 115, Box: Personal Correspondence 4, Folder 5: Letters to Mother and Dad, 1939–1950.

58. David McCullough, *The Greater Journey: Americans in Paris* (New York: Simon & Schuster, 2011) Kindle edition.

59. Bonner, *Iconoclast,* 88 (see chap. 2, n. 37).

60. JPM to Francis McGovern and Lottie Brown, March 28, 1949, Papers, MS 115, Box: Personal Correspondence 4, Folder 5: Letters to Mother and Dad, 1939–1950.

61. Ibid., April 3, 1949, Papers, MS 115, Box: Personal Correspondence 4, Folder 5: Letters to Mother and Dad, 1939–1950.

62. Ibid., May 19, 1949, Papers, MS 115, Box: Personal Correspondence 4, Folder 5: Letters to Mother and Dad, 1939–1950.

63. Ibid. (to May 19).

64. Ibid. (to May 25).

65. Ibid., May 25, 1949, Papers, MS 115, Box: Personal Correspondence 4, Folder 5: Letters to Mother and Dad, 1939–1950.

66. Ibid. (to May 25).

67. Abraham Levinson, "Medallions and plaques of interest to pediatricians," *American Journal of Disabled Children* 62 (1941), 159. Levinson points out that early Egyptian, Greek and Roman coins, which bore the likenesses of emperors or figures of deities, may be considered the forerunners of the medallion. Medical medallions, while not made for monetary use, are special art and date to the fifteenth century, when Piscan, a sculptor in northern Italy, made the first portrait medallion. They typically show a human or symbolic figure in bas-relief on their face (obverse), and the date of issue and other information on the back (reverse).

68. JPM to Francis McGovern and Lottie Brown, May 28, 1949, Papers, MS 115, Box: Personal Correspondence 4, Folder 5: Letters to Mother and Dad, 1939–1950.

69. T. E. C. Jr., "L'Hôpital des Enfants-Malades, The World's First Children's Hospital, Founded in Paris in 1802," *Pediatrics* 67, no. 5 (May 1981): 670.

70. Alex Sakula, "R. T. H. Laënnec 1781–1826: His life and Work: A Bicentenary Appreciation," *Thorax* 36 (1981): 81–90.

71. Joe Sigler, "Dr. John P. McGovern Receives French National Order of Merit," press release, June 1990, Papers, MS 115, Series 7, Box: 9, Folder 9.34, News Releases, 1988–1992, Folder 2.

72. JPM to Francis McGovern and Lottie Brown, May 28, 1949, Papers, MS 115, Box: Personal Correspondence 4, Folder 5: Letters to Mother and Dad, 1939–1950.

73. Ibid.

74. William Osler, *Aequanimitas,* 210 (see chap. 2, n. 10).

75. "History," *George Washington University,* accessed February 9, 2013, http://www.gwu.edu/history.

76. Del Quentin Wilber, *Rawhide Down: The Near Assassination of Ronald Reagan* (New York: Henry Holt, 2011).

77. Doris H. Merritt, contribution to *Appreciations,* 117–18.

78. Hazel Chumley, contribution to *Appreciations,* 106.

79. Merritt, contribution to *Appreciations,* 118.

80. Ibid., 117.

81. Chumley, contribution to *Appreciations,* 107.

82. Donald J. Fernbach, contribution to *Appreciations,* 109.

83. Reginald S. Lourie, contribution to *Appreciations,* 112.

84. Merritt, contribution to *Appreciations,* 121.

85. Lourie, contribution to *Appreciations,* 112.

86. *1970–1971 Annual Report of the John and Mary R. Markle Foundation* (John and Mary R. Markle Foundation: November 1971), 91.

87. John and Mary R. Markle Foundation Records (1960–1994), Finding Aid, Organizational History of Markle Scholarship, Rockefeller Foundation Archives, Rockefeller Archive Center, Sleepy Hollow, New York.

88. Ibid.

89. Ibid.

90. "Francis McGovern, Physician, Is Dead: Ex-Head of Garfield Hospital in Washington Had Been an Advisor to Selective Service," *New York Times*, July 29, 1951.

91. "Lilly Gives Grants to Washington U.," *Washington Post* (undated), Papers, MS 115, Box: Scrapbook 1, 1939–1962, Folder 10: 1953. The article notes two grants received totaling $10,250. Both grants were overseen by McGovern at George Washington University's Gallinger Municipal Hospital.

92. Chumley, contribution to *Appreciations*, 106.

93. JPM to Wilburt C. Davison, May 27, 1952, Papers, MS 115, Series 7, Box 1, Folder 1: Correspondence with Davison 1945–1962.

94. Ibid.

95. Wilburt C. Davison to JPM, July 11, 1952, Papers, MS 115, Box: Davison 1, Folder 5: Davison Correspondence with McGovern 1946–1955.

96. Ibid., July 9, 1952, Papers, MS 115, Series 7, Box 1, Folder 1: Correspondence with Davison 1945–1962.

97. John A. Washington (chairman of the executive committee of the medical staff at George Washington University) to JPM, April 5, 1953, Papers, MS 115, Box: Scrapbook 1, 1939–1962, Folder 10: 1953.

98. JPM to Wilburt C. Davison, June 10, 1954, Papers, MS 115, Series 7, Box 1, Folder 1: Correspondence with Davison 1945–1962.

99. Wilburt C. Davison to JPM, January 19, 1954, Papers, MS 115, Box: Davison 1, Folder 5: Davison Correspondence with McGovern 1946–1955.

100. John Salvaggio, *New Orleans' Charity Hospital: A Story of Physicians, Politics, and Poverty* (Baltimore: Johns Hopkins University Press, 2002), xiii.

101. Ned Sublette, *The World That Made New Orleans: From Spanish Silver to Congo Square* (Chicago: Lawrence Hill, 2008), Kindle edition.

102. Salvaggio, *New Orleans' Charity Hospital*, 11–12.

103. Ibid., 72.

104. H. J. Herring (dean of men at Duke University) to JPM, June 27, 1939, Papers, MS 115, Box: Scrapbook 1, 1939–1962, Folder 1: 1939.

105. John S. Fordtran, contribution to *Appreciations*, 140.

106. James L. Bridges, contribution to *Appreciations*, 137.

107. Salvaggio, *New Orleans' Charity Hospital*, 125.

108. Charity Hospital, *Charity Hospital Annual Board Report 1934–1935*, 29, http://www.tulane.edu/~mates/CHR/CHR1934–1935.pdf; and Charity Hospital, *Charity Hospital Annual Board Report 1937–1939*, 27, 43, http://www.tulane.edu/~mates/CHR/CHR1937–1939.pdf.

109. Salvaggio, *New Orleans' Charity Hospital,* 180.

110. William Osler, *A Way of Life and Selected Writings of Sir William Osler* (New York: Dover, 1951), 249.

111. Hans Weill, Morton M. Ziskind, Richard C. Dickerson, and Vincent J. Derbes, "Epidemic Asthma in New Orleans," *Journal of the American Medical Association* 190, no. 9 (November 30, 1964): 77–78.

112. JPM to Wilburt C. Davison, May 25, 1955, Papers, MS 115, Series 7, Box 1, Folder 1: Correspondence with Davison 1945–1962.

113. Ibid., July 29, 1955, Papers, MS 115, Series 7, Box 1, Folder 1: Correspondence with Davison 1945–1962.

114. JPM to Lottie Brown, July 9, 1955, Papers, MS 115, Box: Personal 4, Folder 7: Jack's letters to Mother 1955–1959.

115. Osler, *Aequanimitas,* 204.

116. JPM to Wilburt C. Davison, July 29, 1955, Papers, MS 115, Series 7, Box 1, Folder 1: Correspondence with Davison 1945–1962.

117. JPM to Lottie Brown, April 14, 1955, Papers, MS 115, Box: Personal Correspondence 4, Folder 7: Jack's letters to Mother 1955–1959.

118. Ibid.

119. S.S. Del Sud Sailing Day Menu—Dinner, August 11, 1955, Papers, MS 115, Box: Personal Correspondence 4, Folder 7: Jack's letters to Mother 1955–1959.

120. JPM to Lottie Brown, April 14, 1955, Papers, MS 115, Box: Personal Correspondence 4, Folder 7: Jack's letters to Mother 1955–1959.

121. "Medicine: Pink Palace of Healing," *Time* (December 13, 1954).

Chapter Four

1. "Facts and Figures," Texas Medical Center, accessed February 9, 2013, http://texasmedicalcenter.org/facts-and-figures/.

2. N. Don Macon, *Monroe Dunaway Anderson, His Legacy: A History of the Texas Medical Center, 50th Anniversary Edition* (Houston: Texas Medical Center, 1994), 65.

3. *It's a Wonderful Life,* directed by Frank Capra (California: Liberty Films,1946).

4. Macon, *Monroe Dunaway Anderson,* 49.

5. Ibid., 27.

6. Erik Larson, *Isaac's Storm* (New York: Crown, 1999), 264–65.

7. Steven Fenberg, *Jesse Jones, Capitalism, and the Common Good* (College Station: Texas A&M University Press, 2011), 61.

8. Macon, *Monroe Dunaway Anderson,* 65.

9. Ibid.

10. Ibid., 71.

11. Ibid., 74.

12. Naomi S. Foster, *A Factual History of George H. Hermann and Hermann Hospital 1925–1975* (Houston: Hermann Hospital Estate, 1975), 1. Copies of this book are located in the John P. McGovern Historical Collections and Research Center Library and the HAM–TMC Library.

13. Garvin Berry and Betty Chapman, "Black Gold Rush: Oilmen Hurried to Humble Field," in *2-Minute Histories of Houston* (Houston: Houston Business Journal Press, 1996), 45.

14. Everett Collier, "George Hermann Remembered," *Houston Chronicle,* May 14, 1951.

15. George Hermann papers, Hermann Hospital Estate Archives. These unprocessed papers are now relocated to the John P. McGovern Historical Collections and Research Center.

16. Nancy Vecera Clark, "George H. Hermann," *New Titles & News,* no. 143 (January 1985): 18, available at the Texas Medical Center Library.

17. Sigmund Byod, "Relative Remembers George Hermann," *Houston Chronicle,* October 2, 1962.

18. Hodge, "A Gift for Giving" (see chap. 1, n. 11).

19. George Hermann papers.

20. Federicka Meiners, *A History of Rice University: The Institute Years, 1907–1963* (Houston: Rice University Historical Commission, 1982), e-book.

21. R. W. Cumley and Joan McCay, eds., *First Twenty Years of the University of Texas M. D. Anderson Hospital and Tumor Institute* (Houston: University of Texas Printing Division, 1964), 13.

22. Macon, *Monroe Dunaway Anderson,* 85.

23. "Vote for the Texas Medical Center," *Houston Post,* December 13, 1943. This was a full-page ad that appeared in Houston's morning newspaper.

24. *The University of Texas Medical Branch at Galveston: A Seventy-Five Year History by the Faculty and Staff* (Austin: University of Texas Press, 1967), 116–17.

25. Walter H. Moursund Sr., *A History of Baylor University College of Medicine 1900—1953* (Houston: Gulf Printing, 1956), 108.

26. Ibid., 117.

27. N. Don Macon, *Clark and the Anderson: A Personal Profile* (Houston: Texas Medical Center, 1976), 12–13.

28. Proceedings at the Dedication of the M. D. Anderson Hospital for Cancer Research, Houston, Texas, February 17, 1944 (Houston: M. D. Anderson Foundation, 1944). A copy of this book is located in the Texas Medical Center Library, Houston.

29. Cumley, *First Twenty Years,* 33.

30. Macon, *Clark and the Anderson,* 189.

31. John Salvaggio, *New Orleans' Charity Hospital,* 147 (see chap. 3, n. 109).

32. Frederick C. Elliott, *The Birth of the Texas Medical Center: A Personal Account* (College Station: Texas A&M University Press, 2004), 31.

33. "Texas Medical Center Welcomes Institutions No. 53 & 54," *Texas Medical Center News,* Nov. 1, 2012.

34. Todd Ackerman, "Q&A with Richard Wainerdi: TMC Research, Care Has Led the World," *Houston Chronicle*, October 28, 2012.

35. Marilyn McAdams Sibley, *The Methodist Hospital of Houston: Serving the World* (Austin: Texas State Historical Association, 1989), 78.

36. Patrick J. Nicholson, *Mr. Jim: The Biography of James Smither Abercrombie* (Houston: Gulf Publishing, 1983).

37. Betsy Parish, *Legacy: 50 Years of Loving Care: Texas Children's Hospital, 1954–2004* (Houston: Elisha Freeman, 2008).

38. Elliott, *Birth of the Texas Medical Center*, 129.

39. Leopold L. Meyer, *The Days of My Life* (Houston: Universal, 1975).

40. Cumley, *First Twenty Years*, 74.

41. JPM, personal conversation with the author, February 1998.

42. Joe Murphy et. al., "Methodology: U. S. News & World Report Best Hospitals 2013–2014," *RTI International*, July 12, 2013.

43. Harvey Grant Taylor, Remembrances and Reflections (Houston: University of Texas Health Science Center, 1991), 7–8.

44. Ibid., 64.

45. Ibid., 106.

46. Ibid., 108.

47. Ibid., 109.

48. Ibid., 139.

49. Grant Taylor to E. J. Bofferding (partner, Cresap, McCormick and Paget Management Consultants), May 25, 1961, Grant Taylor papers, MS 44, Series 1, Box 1: Taylor Series—Personal and Biographical, Folder 8: Correspondence, W. C. Davison, Photograph, Article Reprints, Texas Medical Center Library.

50. Cumley, *First Twenty Years*, 163.

51. Taylor, *Remembrances and Reflections*, 164.

52. William Osler, "The Faith that Heals," *British Medical Journal* 1 (1910): 1470–72.

53. Orville Story, interview by the author, July 24, 2010.

54. Harold H. Bevil, contribution to *Appreciations*, 237 (see intro., n. 1).

55. Walter H. Moursund Sr., "Medicine in Greater Houston 1836–1956" (unpublished manuscript, parts 1 and 2, 1958), 93.

56. Peter B. Kamin, contribution to *Appreciations*, 277–88.

Chapter Five

1. JPM to Lottie Brown, March 6, 1956, Papers, MS 115, Box: Personal Correspondence 4, Folder 7: Jack's letters to Mother 1955–1959.

2. Garvin Berry and Betty Chapman, "Montrose—Pioneer Widow's Land Became Grandest Subdivision," in *2-Minute Histories of Houston* (Houston: Houston Business Journal Press, 1996), 56.

3. Texas Dental College Catalog, 1927, UT Dental Branch Records, IC 9, Series 4, Box 8.

4. Elliott, *Birth of the Texas Medical Center,* 49 (see chap. 4, n. 32).

5. Walter Cronkite, *A Reporter's Life* (New York: Alfred A. Knopf, 1996) 19–20. In 1991 the author wrote a video script celebrating the fiftieth anniversary of M. D. Anderson Cancer Center, with Walter Cronkite agreeing to narrate the script at CBS radio studios in New York City (Black Rock). During that visit and taping session, the author had the opportunity to talk with Cronkite about that reporter's early childhood in Houston, the Texas Dental College, and Fred Elliott—a conversation that is reflected in some of the stories in this book.

6. Berry, "Montrose—Pioneer Widow's Land," in *2-Minute Histories of Houston,* 55.

7. Ibid., 28.

8. Sir Walter Scott, *A Legend of Montrose* (London: Aegypan, 2006).

9. United States Census Bureau, "Texas Dominates List of Fastest-Growing Large Cities since 2010 Census, Census Bureau Reports," press release, June 28, 2012, http://www.census.gov/newsroom/releases/archives/population/cb12-117.html.

10. Ada Holland, contribution to *Appreciations,* 267 (see intro., n. 1).

11. Maxine Mayo, contribution to *Appreciations,* 288.

12. Theodore J. Haywood, contribution to *Appreciations,* 173.

13. Ibid.

14. Orville C. Thomas, contribution to *Appreciations,* 216.

15. Betty Heitman (the Heitman Group) to the president (Ronald Reagan), November 28, 1988, Papers, MS 115, Series 7, Box 13, Folder 22: Correspondence with Betty Heitman 1988–1991; recommendation for Presidential Medal of Freedom.

16. Kathrine G. McGovern, interview by the author, August 18, 2010.

17. JPM to Wilburt C. Davison, December 18, 1961, Papers, MS 115, Series 7, Box 1, Folder 1: Correspondence with Davison 1945–1962.

18. Wilburt C. Davison to Mrs. Joseph McClain Galbreath, March 15, 1962, Papers, MS 115, Series 7, Box 1, Folder 1: Correspondence with Davison 1945–1962.

19. JPM to Wilburt C. Davison, May 25, 1955, Papers, MS 115, Series 7, Box 1, Folder 1: Correspondence with Davison 1945–1962.

20. JPM to Lottie Brown, January 5, 1956, Papers, MS 115, Box: Personal Correspondence 4, Folder 7: Jack's Letters to Mother 1955–1959.

21. Julia Q. Mitchell, e-mail message to the author, November 20, 2012. This communication included a copy of the original Articles of Incorporation of the Texas Allergy Research Foundation (filed September 18, 1961) and a copy of the Certificate of Amendment from the state of Texas office of the secretary of state, George W. Strake Jr., certifying the name change to John P. McGovern Foundation and dated December 5, 1979).

22. Betty Heitman to the president (Ronald Reagan).

23. Theodore Haywood (physician, associate at the McGovern Allergy Clinic), interview by the author, November 18, 2010.

24. Kathrine G. McGovern, interview by the author, September 14, 2012.

Following this meeting the author received a typed summary of Mrs. McGovern's wedding day recollections from December 20, 1961.

25. Ibid., August 18, 2010.

26. Ibid.

27. JPM to Wilburt C. Davison, June 7, 1965, Papers, MS 115, Series 7, Box 1, Folder 7: Correspondence with Wilburt Davison, 1967.

28. William Osler, *Aequanimitas,* 356–57.

29. For a photograph of Senator Lyndon Johnson's reception for the Texas delegation to the White House Conference on Children and Youth in Washington, DC, June 1960, see Papers, MS 115, Box: Scrapbook 1, 1939–1962, Folder 17: 1960.

30. "McGovern Honored by US Surgeon General," *Pulse,* newsletter of the American School Health Association (Bethesda, Maryland), April/May 1980.

31. JPM to Wilburt C. Davison, June 7, 1965, Papers, MS 115, Series 7, Box 1, Folder 3: Correspondence with Wilburt Davison and Jay M. Arena, 1964–1965.

32. Kathrine G. McGovern, interview by the author, August 18, 2010.

33. Mavis P. Kelsey Jr., *Twentieth Century Doctor: House Calls to Space Medicine* (College Station: Texas A&M University Press, 1999), 167.

34. Ibid.

35. Ibid., 174.

36. Ibid., 131.

37. William Henry Kellar and Vaishali J. Patel, *Kelsey-Seybold Clinic: A Legacy of Excellence in Health Care* (Houston, KS Management Services, LLP, 1999), 32.

38. Kelsey, *Twentieth Century Doctor,* 241.

39. JPM to Wilburt C. Davison, March 7, 1971, Papers, MS 115, Series 7, Box 1, Folder 25: Correspondence with Wilburt Davison, 1970–1971.

40. JPM, personal conversation with the author, February 1998.

41. JPM to Friends (all former residents and fellows), June 4, 1973, Papers, MS 115, Box: 20a McGovern Professional, Folder 5: New Clinic Building.

42. Stanley W. Olson to JPM, memorandum, July 1, 1960, Papers, MS 115, Box: Scrapbook 1, 1939–1962, Folder 17: 1960.

43. Thomas M. Daniel, "The History of Tuberculosis," *Respiratory Medicine* 100, no. 11 (2006): 1862–1870.

44. JPM to Wilburt C. Davison, August 16, 1968, Papers, MS 115, Series 7, Box 1, Folder 10: Correspondence with Wilburt Davison, Folder 1 of 2, 1945–1972. In this letter, which responded to an August 12 letter from Davison, McGovern commented that he had not known of the Pirquets' joint suicide and that the information was useful as he had been selected (two years in advance) to give the 1970 Bela Schick Memorial Lecture for the American College of Allergists. He adds that he once met Bela Schick, and (in typical McGovern-the-collector style) had an inscribed photo of him to display in his clinic.

45. American College of Allergy and Immunology, "50th Anniversary Video Script," Steve Campus Productions, Tuckahoe, New York (September 28, 1992),

Papers, MS 115, Box 5: Office Files, Folder 6: American College of Allergists 1989 forward, 4.

46. Ibid., 14–16.

47. Toshiyuki Takai and Hajime Karasuyama, "The Study of Allergy by Japanese Researchers: A Historical Perspective," *International Immunology* 21, no. 12 (2009): 1311–16.

48. JPM and James A. Knight, *Allergy and Human Emotions* (Springfield, Illinois: Charles C Thomas, 2008), vii.

49. Coleman M. Harris, "Allergy and Human Emotions," *Archives of Internal Medicine* 121, no. 3 (1968): 305–6.

50. Mark Jackson, *Allergy: The History of a Modern Malady* (London: Reaktion Books, 2006), 78.

51. Mary Jane Schier, "Allergist—Dr. John P. McGovern of Houston Will Be Installed as President of the American College of Allergists Thursday at the College's Annual Congress in Denver," *Houston Post*, March 28, 1968. A copy of the cited article can be found in Papers, MS 115, Box: Scrapbook 21957–1963/1964–1966, Folder 10: JPM Scrapbook 1968.

52. James A. Murray, contribution to *Appreciations*, 194–95.

53. M. Coleman Harris, contribution to *Appreciations*, 414.

54. Betsy Parish, *Legacy: 50 Years*, 23 (see chap. 4, n. 37).

55. Ibid., 144.

56. Ibid., 143.

57. "Medicine: The Bubble Boy's Lost Battle," *Time*, March 5, 1984, http://www.time.com/time/magazine/article/0,9171,952358,00.html.

58. "The Boy in the Bubble," *PBS American Experience*, produced and directed by Barak Goodman and John Maggio (WGBH Educational Foundation and Ark Media, LLC, 2006).

59. "HIV and AIDS—United States, 1981–2000," *Morbidity and Mortality Weekly Report* 50, no. 21 (June 1, 2001).

60. Taylor H. Grant, *An Historical Resume of the University of Texas Postgraduate School of Medicine* (Houston: University of Texas, 1958), i.

61. Ibid., iii.

62. Minutes of the University of Texas Board of Regents Meeting (Austin: University of Texas, September 29, 1950), 6.

63. Kelsey, *Twentieth Century Doctor*, 233 (see chap. 4, n. 3).

64. James S. Olson, *Making Cancer History: Disease & Discovery at the University of Texas M. D. Anderson Cancer Center* (Baltimore: Johns Hopkins University Press, 2009), 77.

65. Ibid., 76.

66. Taylor, *Remembrances and Reflections*,167–68 (see chap. 4, n. 43).

67. Glenn Knotts, personal conversation with the author, February 3, 1994.

68. Charles G. Roland et al., "William Osler Commemorative Issue," special

issue, *Journal of the American Medical Association* 210, no. 12 (December 22, 1969): 2213–71.

69. JPM to Wilburt C. Davison, August 8, 1968, Papers, MS 115, Series 7, Box. 1, Folder 22: Correspondence with Wilburt Davison, 1968.

70. O. C. Thomas and T. J. Haywood to McGovern Allergy Clinic staff, memorandum, April 23, 1969, Papers, MS 115, Box: Scrapbook 3, 1968–2000, Folder 5: 1969.

71. Wilburt C. Davison to JPM, September 25, 1970, Papers, MS 115, Series 7, Box 1, Folder 10: Correspondence with Wilburt Davison, Folder 1 of 2, 1945–1972.

72. Hodge, "A Gift for Giving" (see chap. 1, n. 11).

73. Wilburt C. Davison, transcript of oral history interview by Frank Rounds, 1969, 139–40, Papers, MS 115, Box: Davison 4, Folder 1: Davison Oral History.

74. Ibid.

75. Ibid.

76. Hodge, "A Gift for Giving."

77. Kathrine G. McGovern, interview by the author, August 18, 2010.

78. Obituary, "Orville Leroy Story," *Houston Chronicle*, May 30, 2012.

79. Orville Story, interview by the author, July 24, 2010.

80. Ibid.

81. Ibid.

82. Orville C. Thomas to Friends of McGovern Allergy Clinic, May 12, 1981, Papers, MS 115, Box 6: Professional: Festschrift continued; McGovern Correspondence; Texas Medical, Folder 12: Dr. Thomas's letter re: JPM dinner 5/5/1981.

83. Roger Bulger, e-mail message to author, September 20, 2012.

84. Harold Y. Vanderpool, review of *Physician and Philosopher: The Philosophical Foundation of Medicine: Essays*, by Dr. Edwund Pellegrino, ed. Roger J. Bulger and JPM, *New England Journal of Medicine* 347 (September 19, 2002): 952–53; and Roger Bulger, "The Quest for the Therapeutic Organization," *Journal of the American Medical Association* 283, no. 18 (May 10, 2000): 2431–33.

85. Roger J. Bulger, *Healing America: Hope, Mercy, Justice and Autonomy in the American Health Care System* (Westport, Connecticut: Prospecta Press, 2010), xiv.

86. Hodge, "A Gift for Giving."

87. JPM to Francis McGovern and Lottie Brown, April 10, 1943, Papers, MS 115, Box: Personal Correspondence 4, Folder 5: Letters to Mother and Dad, 1939–1950.

88. Ibid. to Lottie Brown, March 22, 1940, Papers, MS 115, Box: Personal Correspondence 4, Folder 5: Letters to Mother and Dad, 1939–1950.

89. Betty Heitman to the president (Ronald Reagan).

90. Betty Ford to the president (George H. Bush), March 5, 1991, Papers, MS 115, Series 7, Box 13, Folder 18: Correspondence with Betty Ford about Her Recommendation for Presidential Medal of Freedom.

91. Betty Heitman to the president (Ronald Reagan).

92. Hodge, "A Gift for Giving."

Chapter Six

1. Rotary Club of Houston, President Derek S. Munger, *Distinguished Citizen Award Gala Honoring John P. McGovern, M. D.,* September 13, 2001 (Houston: Rotary Club of Houston, 2001).

2. President George H. Bush, "Rotary Club of Houston Celebration of John P. McGovern as Houston's 2001 Distinguished Citizen of the Year," remarks recorded for presentation at the Hyatt Regency Hotel, Houston, September 13, 2001.

3. Charles A. LeMaistre, remarks at the celebration.

4. JPM, honoree's remarks at the celebration.

5. Event program for the forty-first annual meeting of the American Osler Society, Philadelphia, May 1–4, 2011.

6. Ibid.

7. JPM and Chester R. Burns, eds., *Humanism in Medicine* (Springfield, Illinois: Charles C. Thomas, 1980), xii.

8. Wilburt C. Davison to JPM, October 9, 1967, Papers, MS 115, Series 7, Box 1, Folder 7: Correspondence with Wilburt Davison 1967.

9. JPM to Wilburt C. Davison, October 31, 1967, Papers, MS 115, Series 7, Box 1, Folder 7: Correspondence with Wilburt Davison 1967.

10. Wilburt C. Davison to JPM, December 1, 1969, Papers, MS 115, Box: Davison 1, Folder 6: Davison Correspondence with McGovern 1960–1972.

11. Alfred Henderson to JPM, April 9, 1970, Papers, MS 115, Box: American Osler Society 2b, Folder 5: AOS Correspondence 1968–1974.

12. Alfred R. Henderson and JPM, "The American Osler Society: Its Occasion for Being and Its Origin," *Southern Medical Journal* 67, no. 10 (October 1974): 1209–11.

13. Charles G. Roland et al., *William Osler Commemorative Issue,* 2213–71 (see chap. 5, n. 68).

14. Jeremiah A. Barondess, Charles G. Roland, and JPM, eds., *The Persisting Osler: : Selected Transactions of the American Osler Society, 1991–2000,* vol. 3 (Malabar, Florida: Krieger, 2002), 189–201. See especially the chapter by Charles G. Roland, "The Formative Years of the American Osler Society."

15. William B. Bean and JPM, "Osler's Influence on William Bean," *Archives of Internal Medicine* 134, no. 5 (November 1974): 844–45.

16. Barondess, *The Persisting Osler, 191.*

17. JPM to Willard E. Goodwin, December 9, 1969, Papers, MS 115, Box: American Osler Society 2b, Folder 5: AOS Correspondence 1968–1974. This is the letter McGovern and Henderson sent to prospective members of the new organization.

18. Symposium Program of "Humanism in Medicine: As Portrayed by the Life of Sir William Osler," April 21–22, 1970, Flagship Hotel, Galveston, Texas, Papers, MS 115, Box 6, Folder 19.

19. Event Program for the First Annual Meeting of the American Osler Society, April 1, 1971, the Denver Hilton, Papers, MS 115, Box 6, Folder 19.

20. Alfred R. Henderson, "Comments on the American Osler Society and an Introduction of William Bean," *Hopkins Medical Journal* 129, no. 6 (December 1971): 343–45.

21. Barondess *The Persisting Osler,* 189.

22. William Osler, "The Old Humanities and the New Science" (presidential address delivered before the Classical Association, Oxford, May 16, 1919), *British Medical Journal* 2 (July 1919): 1–7.

23. William Regelson, "The Weakening of the Oslerian Tradition: The Changing Emphasis in Departments of Medicine," *Journal of the American Medical Association* 239, no. 4 (January 23, 1978).

24. "Five-Year Report on the McGovern Center for Humanities & Ethics" (Houston: John P. McGovern, M.D. Center for Humanities and Ethics, University of Texas Health Science Center at Houston, 2010).

25. Lynn M. Alperin, "The John P. McGovern Academy of Oslerian Medicine: The First Ten Years" (Galveston: John P. McGovern Academy of Oslerian Medicine, 2012).

26. To access the minutes and get a feeling for their scope, see "Annual Report of the National Library of Medicine Programs and Services, Fiscal Year 1973," US Department of Health, Education, and Welfare, Public Health Service, publication 74–286, 6. Note that the number of board members has varied over the years. For the names of members in 1974, when McGovern was chair, see the minutes of the 47th meeting of the Board of Regents of the National Library of Medicine, Department of Health, Education and Welfare, March 21–22, 1974, at Florida State University in Tallahassee, http://www.nlm.nih.gov/hmd/manuscripts/nlm archives/bor/1974.pdf.

27. Martin M. Cummings to JPM, January 23, 1970, Papers, MS 115, Box: Scrapbook 3, Folder 7: 1969.

28. Wyndham D. Miles, *A History of The National Library of Medicine—The National's Treasury of Medical Knowledge* (Bethesda, Maryland: U.S. Department of Health and Human Services, Public Health Service, National Institutes of Health publication 85–1904, 1985), 355.

29. Michele Lyons, *70 Acres of Science: The NIH Moves to Bethesda* (Bethesda, Maryland: US Department of Health and Human Services, Public Health Service, National Institutes of Health, 2006), http://history.nih.gov/research/downloads /70acresofscience.pdf

30. Miles, *A History of the National Library of Medicine,* 347.

31. *Hirshhorn Museum: Hearings on HR 15121, before the Subcommittee of Public Buildings and Grounds of the Committee on Public Works,* 89th Congress, 2nd session (1966).

32. Aaron Myers, "All Eyes on the Hirshhorn, but It Wasn't Always Pretty (or

Round)," *Ghosts of DC* (blog), March 22, 2012, http://ghostsofdc.org/2012/03/22/all-eyes-on-the-hirshhorn-but-it-wasnt-always-pretty-or-round/#1.

33. Wilburt C. Davison to JPM, September 25, 1970, Papers, MS 115, Series 7, Box 1, Folder 10: Correspondence with Wilburt Davison, Folder 1 of 2, 1945–1972.

34. William D. Mayer, "Martin M. Cummings, M.D.: A Remarkable Man Retires with a Truly Remarkable Legacy," *Bulletin of the Medical Library Association* 72, no. 1 (January 1984): 35.

35. Minutes of the 47th Meeting of the Board of Regents of the National Library of Medicine (see n. 26 above).

36. "Annual Report of the National Library of Medicine Programs and Services, Fiscal Year 1973," 6; and Mayer, "Martin M. Cummings," 35.

37. Mayer, "Martin M. Cummings," 35.

38. Williams & Wilkins Co. v. United States, 487 F. 2d 1345 (Ct. Cl. 1973), affirmed by an equally divided court, 420 US 376 (1975).

39. Martin M. Cummings to JPM, November 15, 1967, Papers, MS 115, Box: Davison 3, Folder 3: Davison—Articles about Him.

40. Fielding H. Garrison, *John Shaw Billings: A Memoir* (New York: G. P. Putnam's Sons, 1915), 221; Wyndham D. Miles, *A History of The National Library of Medicine;* and James H. Cassedy, *John Shaw Billings: Science and Medicine in the Gilded Age* (Bethesda, Maryland: Xlibris, 2009).

41. Joyce Marson, "John Shaw Billings as a Bibliographer," *Bulletin of the Medical Library Association* 57, no. 4 (October 1969): 380.

42."Factsheet: IndexCat," National Library of Medicine, last modified May 17, 2012, http://www.nlm.nih.gov/pubs/factsheets/indexcat.html.

43. Stephen J. Greenberg and Patricia E. Gallagher, "The Great Contribution: Index Medicus, Index-Catalogue, and IndexCat," *Journal of the Medical Library Association* 97, no. 2 (April 2009): 108–13.

44. Stephen B. Greenberg, "Osler-Web-Rendezvous: Impact of the Information Explosion on Medical Education," *Transactions of the American Clinical and Climatological Association* 119 (2008), 245–61.

45. Martin M. Cummings to JPM, November 15, 1967, Papers, MS 115, Box: Davison 3, Folder 3: Davison—Articles about Him.

46. Stephen B. Greenberg, "Osler-Web-Rendezvous."

47. *Houston Academy of Medicine–Texas Medical Center Library, Annual Report: FY 2011–12* (Houston: HAM–TMC, 2013).

48. M. J. Figard (curator of the McGovern Rare Books Collection, HAM–TMC Library), e-mail to the author, September 19, 2012.

49. Elizabeth White (retired director of the HAM–TMC Library Rare Books and Archives Collections), interview by the author, September 6, 2011.

50. Renee C. Lee, "Medical Pioneer Tackles New Projects as He Nears 100," *Houston Chronicle,* September 30, 2012.

51. Mary Sit-DuVall, "Dr. Mavis Kelsey Looks Back: Building a Medical

Dynasty," *Houston Chronicle,* July 6, 1999. Kelsey-Seybold had hoped to renovate McGovern's building and integrate it into their campus design but eventually decided to raze it instead. Contractors reported they had a devil of a time tearing the structure down as McGovern had built it strong enough to withstand additional floors if needed.

52. Julia Q. Mitchell, e-mail to the author, July 7, 2012.

53. "McGovern Health Museum 2011: By the Numbers," Fact Sheet (Houston: John P. McGovern Museum of Health & Medical Science, May 2012).

Chapter Seven

1. William Osler, "The Student Life," in *Aequanimitas,* 397–98 (see chap. 2, n. 10).

2. Charles G. Roland, "The Infamous William Osler," *Journal of the American Medical Association* 193, no. 6 (1965): 436.

3. William B. Bean, "Osler, Trollope, and the Fixed Period," *Transactions of the American Clinical and Climatological Association* 78, (1967): 242–48.

4. Harvey Cushing, *The Life of Sir William Osler,* 682 (see chap. 2, n. 5).

5. Hilda Pope Willett, contribution to *Appreciations,* 53 (see intro., n. 1).

6. Orville Story, interview by the author, July 24, 2010.

7. "Distinguished Alumni 1999: Glenn R. Knotts," Purdue University College of Pharmacy, accessed March 18, 2013, http://www.pharmacy.purdue.edu/advancement/honors/distinguished/1999_knotts.php.

8. Glenn Knotts, personal conversation with the author, March 2001.

9. "Gun Used in Shooting Believed Found," *Houston Chronicle,* July 23, 1996.

10. Glenn Knotts, personal conversation with the author, June 13, 2002.

11. Lynwood Abram, "Deaths: Glenn Knotts, 68, Instrumental Force behind Eye Center," *Houston Chronicle,* January 16, 2003.

12. Glenn Knotts, personal conversation with the author, June 13, 2002.

13. Julia Q. Mitchell, interview by the author, August 25, 2010.

14. Ibid.

15. Gail Glass (office staff member for McGovern), interview by the author, October 12, 2010.

16. Ibid.

17. Bill McLemore (laboratory supervisor, McGovern Allergy Clinic), interview by the author, November 18, 2010.

18. Ibid.

19. Gay Collette (grants manager, McGovern Foundation), interview by the author, October 12, 2010.

20. Ibid.

21. William Osler, *Aequanimitas,* 356–57.

22. Julia Q. Mitchell, interview by the author, August 25, 2010.

23. Gay Collette, interview by the author, October 12, 2010.

24. Ibid.

25. Ibid.

26. Jeanette Mattiza (investments broker for McGovern), telephone interview by the author, January 25, 2011.

27. JPM to unnamed individual, March 8, 1972, Papers, MS 115, Box: McGovern Professional 33, Folder 6: McGovern, John P.—personal 1972.

28. Orville Story, interview by the author, July 24, 2010.

29. Ibid.

30. Kathrine G. McGovern, interview by the author, August 18, 2010.

31. Billy F. Andrews, "A Privileged Friendship with John P. McGovern," *Oslerian* 8, no. 2 (2007): 5–6.

32. Notable among the obituaries are these: Jeremy Pearce, "John McGovern, 85, Allergist, Investor and Philanthropist, Dies," *New York Times,* June 11, 2007; "John P. McGovern, M.D., 1921–2007," *Houston Chronicle,* June 5, 2007; and Dale Lezon and Todd Ackerman, "Doctor Became Known for Giving," *Houston Chronicle,* June 11, 2007.

Bibliography of Books by John P. McGovern, MD

Mandel, W., J. H. Thomas, C. T. Carman, and J. P. McGovern. *Bibliography on Sarcoidosis: 1876–1963*. Washington, DC: US Department of Health, Education, and Welfare, 1964.

McGovern, J. P., and J. A. Knight. *Allergy and Human Emotions*. Springfield, Illinois: Charles C. Thomas, 1967.

McGovern, J. P., ed. *A Way of Life*. By Sir William Osler. Springfield, Illinois: Charles C. Thomas, 1969.

McGovern, J. P., and C. G. Roland. *Wm. Osler: The Continuing Education*. Springfield, Illinois: Charles C. Thomas, 1969.

Stewart, G. T., and J. P. McGovern. *Penicillin Allergy: Clinical and Immunological Aspects*. Springfield, Illinois: Charles C. Thomas, 1970.

Swineford, O., Jr. Edited by J. P. McGovern. *Asthma and Hay Fever*. Springfield, Illinois: Charles C. Thomas, 1971.

McGovern, J. P., and C. R. Burns. *Humanism in Medicine*. Springfield, Illinois: Charles C. Thomas, 1974.

Knotts, G. R., and McGovern, J. P. *School Health Problems*. Springfield, Illinois: Charles C. Thomas, 1975.

McGovern, J. P., ed. *Davison Memorial Addresses*. Austin: University of Texas Press, 1976.

Nation, E. F., C. G. Roland, and J. P. McGovern. *An Annotated Checklist of Osleriana*. Kent, Ohio: Kent State University Press, 1976.

McGovern, J. P., M. H. Smolensky, and A. Reinberg. *Chronobiology in Allergy and Immunology*. Springfield, Illinois: Charles C Thomas, 1977.

Arena, J., and J. P. McGovern, eds. *Davison of Duke—His Reminiscences*. Durham: Duke University Medical Center, 1980.

Nation, E. F., and J. P. McGovern, eds. *Student and Chief: The Osler-Camac Correspondence*. Pasadena: Castle Press, 1980.

Smolensky, M. H., A. Reinberg, and J. P. McGovern. *Recent Advances in the Chronobiology of Allergy and Immunology.* Oxford: Pergamon Press, 1980.

Barondess, J. A., C. G. Roland, and J. P. McGovern, eds. *The Persisting Osler: Selected Transactions of the American Osler Society, 1991–2000.* Vol. 3 Baltimore, Ohio: University Park Press, 1985.

McGovern, J. P., and C. G. Roland, eds. *The Collected Essays of Sir William Osler.* Vol. 1. Birmingham: Classics of Medicine Library, 1985.

McGovern, J. P., and C. G. Roland, eds. *The Collected Essays of Sir William Osler.* Vol. 2. Birmingham: Classics of Medicine Library, 1985.

McGovern, J. P., and C. G. Roland, eds. *The Collected Essays of Sir William Osler.* Vol. 3. Birmingham: Classics of Medicine Library, 1985.

Van Eys, J., and J. P. McGovern, eds. *The Doctor as a Person.* Springfield, Illinois: Charles C. Thomas, 1988.

Starck, P. L., and J. P. McGovern, eds. *The Hidden Dimension of Illness: Human Suffering.* New York: National League for Nursing Press, 1992.*

Taylor, H. G., N. D. Macon, and J. P. McGovern, eds. *Remembrances & Reflections.* Houston: University of Texas Health Science Center Press, 1992.

McGovern, J. P., and R. L. DuPont. *A Bridge to Recovery—An Introduction to 12-Step Programs.* Washington, DC: American Psychiatric Press, 1994.

Boutwell, B., and McGovern, J. P.: *Conversation with a Medical School—The University of Texas-Houston Medical School, 1970–2000.* Houston: University of Texas-Houston Health Science Center, 1999.†

Nation, E. F., C. G. Roland, and J. P. McGovern. *An Annotated Checklist of Osleriana.* Vol. 1. Kent, Ohio: Kent State University Press, 1976. Rev. ed., Montreal: Osler Library, McGill University, 2000.

Nation, E. F., C. G. Roland, and J. P. McGovern. *An Annotated Checklist of Osleriana.* Vol. 2. Kent, Ohio: Kent State University Press, 1976. Rev. ed., Montreal: Osler Library, McGill University, 2000.

Bulger, R. J., and J. P. McGovern, eds. *Physician Philosopher: The Philosophical Foundation of Medicine: Essays.* By Dr. Edmund Pellegrino. Charlottesville, Virginia: Carden Jennings, 2001.

*1992 Book of the Year Award, *American Journal of Nursing*

†2000 Matrix Award, first place

Index